T0129812

# The Epilepsy Book:
# A Companion for Patients

Thalia Valeta

# The Epilepsy Book:
# A Companion for Patients

Optimizing Diagnosis and Treatment

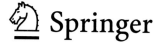 Springer

Thalia Valeta
First Neurology and Psychiatry Clinic
University of Athens, Aeginition Hospital
Athens
Greece

Department of Clinical Neurophysiology
and Epilepsies
St. Thomas' Hospital
London
UK

The cover of the book is based on a drawing by the author.

ISBN 978-3-319-87132-5        ISBN 978-3-319-61679-7    (eBook)
DOI 10.1007/978-3-319-61679-7

Printed on acid-free paper

This Springer imprint is published by Springer Nature
The registered company is Springer International Publishing AG
The registered company address is: Gewerbestrasse 11, 6330 Cham, Switzerland

# Foreword

I have had the profound privilege of caring for people with epilepsy over the course of my career. Time and time again, I personally witnessed the toll that epilepsy could exact on virtually every aspect of a person's life and on their family. Much of this toll was independent of whether seizures were controlled. What became clear was that epilepsy care needed to evolve beyond a singular focus on seizure control to more holistically enabling people with epilepsy to live up to their full potential.

Of central importance to achieving this new paradigm is effective communication between persons with epilepsy, their families, and their healthcare providers to enhance patient self-empowerment and improve health outcomes. This communication must respect cultural sensitivities and address the unfavorable attitudes towards people with epilepsy in society that perpetuate stigma.

Epilepsy and its effects on lives are complicated topics and those who are newly diagnosed or who do not respond to treatments are particularly in need of accurate information that they can understand and which is presented in a clear, nonjudgmental and yet encouraging format. This information is most useful when it also helps patients and their families to ask the right questions and to access a wide range of credible resources to supplement their knowledge and bolster their self-confidence.

This wonderful book achieves all of these goals. It provides information for people with epilepsy and their families on a wide range of important topics including an overview of epilepsy, seizures, epileptic syndromes, sudden unexpected death in epilepsy, comorbidities, nonepileptic seizures, special considerations for women, psychosocial aspects, safety considerations, and diagnostic tests. Also covered are treatments ranging from antiepileptic drugs to integrative approaches to diets to psychological therapies, including "Metamyth"©, an innovative, neuroscience-informed, culturally sensitive blending of the arts in a theater-based setting to facilitate healing and self-empowerment.

Within each chapter, sections are identified by questions that patients with epilepsy and their families are likely to ask their healthcare providers. There are also recommendations that further help with communication as well as useful links and references. The last chapter is a comprehensive compilation of resources that are fully described.

The doctor-patient relationship, when based on a partnership, is vitally important for charting a path to healing. This book will be your guide and inspiration to stay on course.

Boston, MA, USA                                                               Steven C. Schachter, M.D.

# Praises Abridged

This book is a gem, an "all-in-one" and "must-have" indispensable guide for people with epilepsy and their families. Thalia Valeta considers all aspects of their medical and psychosocial needs with reader—friendly reliable information and recommendations.

C. P. Panayiotopoulos, M.D., Ph.D., F.R.C.P.

Thalia Valeta has pioneered the field of Dramatherapy and Epilepsy. Her book provides essential information in what the patients with epilepsy should know to optimize diagnosis and treatment.

Dr. A. Covanis, M.D., D.C.H., Ph.D., Child Neurologist President IBE

Using the approach of "Metamyth" © which is unique to Thalia Valeta, the book seeks to open up dialogue about epilepsy and demonstrates a transparency of communication. It builds a bridge between medicine and psychology through the applied field of neurology.

Professor Sue Jennings Ph.D.

This book reveals creative and compassionate ways to work with people suffering from epilepsy. "Metamyth" © is innovative, dynamic, and evidencing humane.

J Quennell Jungian Psychotherapist
Head of Dramatherapy London School of Speech and Drama

# Acknowledgments

This book would not be possible without the patients who have impressed and inspired me by confiding to me their questions and problems. This put me in the position to respond and help as a practicing psychotherapist/dramatherapist, also filling in the need for an emotionally literate approach to therapy with "Metamyth"©, a psychological therapy through the arts for people with epilepsy.

I would like to thank my husband Prof. C. P. Panayiotopoulos, who has been my private tutor on epilepsy for 40 years and for his valuable assistance with advice, on the medical part of the book.

Prof. Steven C. Schachter for writing the Foreword for my book.

Dr. A. Covanis for providing the opportunity to complete my research on the parental reactions and needs of children with epilepsy at Agia Sophia Children's Hospital in Athens.

Neurologists and Psychiatrists in the First Neurology and Psychiatry Clinic at the University of Athens for referring patients to the "Metamyth"©/Dramatherapy Clinic at the Aeginition Hospital Athens.

Dr. M. Koutroumanidis, Consultant Neurologist at St. Thomas' Hospital for offering me the position of Honorary Lecturer and Researcher in the Epilepsy Clinic at St. Thomas'.

My son who has encouraged me by being so perfect himself and my lovely daughter for her love.

Jocelyn Quenell, Dramatherapist and Jungian Analyst, Leader of the Sesame program at the London School of Speech and Drama, for her valuable advice.

My teacher Prof. Sue Jennings, one of the founders of Dramatherapy, for supervising my work.

Finally Joanna Bolesworth, Melissa Morton, William Curtis, and Andre Tournois at Springer Publishing for offering me to write, *The Epilepsy Book: A Companion for Patients*.

May 28, 2017                                        Thalia Valeta, B.A., M.A., HPC reg.

# Contents

# About the Author

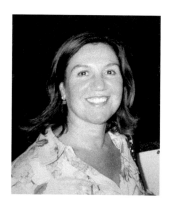

**Thalia Valeta, B.A., M.A., H.P.C** is a dramatherapist, actress, and writer. She is the founder and director of "Metamyth" © Therapy through the Arts, a psychological treatment which she practices with people who have epilepsy and other neurological or psychiatric disorders. Her contributions also include the psychosocial issues, parental reactions, and needs of children with epilepsy. She has published in significant journals and books. She is an activist in the Global campaign against stigma.

Thalia is an Honorary Researcher and Lecturer in St. Thomas' hospital, London, and works as a therapist in the First Neurology and Psychiatry Clinic at the University of Athens. She gives "Metamyth" © workshops in museums and art centers internationally.

# Introduction

This book is the product of my involvement for 17 years with people who have epilepsy, research in the field of epilepsy, working as a psychotherapist/dramatherapist and lecturing on this subject of my interest.

**The Story** My motivation for exploring the subject of epilepsy has been informed by two areas of my professional and personal experience.

Firstly, I was working at a clinic responsible for the treatment of epilepsy. In this role, I found that patients had a very real need to talk about their experiences and confided in me their suffering. This meant that I was being informally positioned in the role of counsellor which alerted me to the potentially unmet psychological needs in the delivery of services. I was also then working as an actress, and this informed the specific choice to develop my knowledge and expertise in the field of Dramatherapy.

Secondly, as a consequence of working in a clinic with physicians specializing in the treatment of epilepsy, I have been exposed to a great deal of related international research. From my own perspective, it became clear to me that they were very serious limits in the approach of the medical model and that epilepsy can have a profound emotional impact on the whole family surrounding the person or those affected. The need for an active, emotionally literate approach to therapy that focused on imagination and the relationship between client and therapist was clear to me.

My first degree in media and cultural studies and my work at the arts desk of newspapers reviewing theatre plays, on the principle that the private can become public for the benefit of society, have helped me to pursue my interests and I conducted a research project presented in Chap. 24, which involved designing a questionnaire for families. My aim was to give the opportunity to parents of children who have epilepsy to express their feelings and identify their needs. The results showed that children and adolescents with epilepsy and their families need more than medical therapeutic support to obtain an acceptable quality of life. This was published and caught the attention of researchers working as medical specialists in this area.

This encouraged me to learn more about psychotherapy, dance, alternative medicine and complementary therapies so as to consider what these paradigms and approaches to treatment have to offer. In particular, I was interested in the significance of the neurobiological approach to psychotherapy and the body and emotion for both the individual suffering with epilepsy and the impact on those who witness the epileptic seizures.

I had already begun my experience of theatre and dance and the philosophy of complementary medicines and was presenting this with the name "Metamyth"©. Originally, I used "Metamyth"© as a technique to help actors play their part. It enabled them to explore aspects of their personality that were appropriate to the role they were about to play.

Epilepsy patients and my will to help them in an effective way were always uppermost in my mind. This is when I was inspired and decided to train as a Dramatherapist in order to be able to offer psychological support to patients who have epilepsy in a scientific and professional way. In my research, I have found no reports on Dramatherapy with people who have epilepsy and I am pioneering this area of research since 2009 with my thesis, The Potential of Dramatherapy in the Treatment of Epilepsy.

**The Book** This book is to inform patients about their condition, help them to optimize their diagnosis, treatment and management and contribute to a better understanding of their epilepsy. Thus, its purpose is to provide patients with epilepsy and their families with appropriate guidance and be a companion in their inquest for the correct diagnosis, management and personal fulfilment. This book provides answers to commonly asked questions about epilepsy, dispel uncertainties and fears, minimize the possibility of misdiagnosis and mismanagement and encourage those diagnosed with epilepsy to become strong advocates in their medical care.

The book aims to bring, together with the medical model, psychological approaches as parallel treatments to help alleviate the symptoms and comorbidities of epilepsy and support the patients towards a good quality of life making use of their full potential.

Because Epilepsy has more coexisting physical and psychological symptoms, than any other disease, it can be interpreted as both a physiological process and a psychic one. This book provides extensive information and explanations on medical issues and psychological disturbances of patients with epilepsy. As you will see, in many chapters a psychological treatment is needed to take care of the psychological needs of people with epilepsy, as well as the medical science which looks after the physical body. This principle, you will find, runs through the whole book.

As I am a psychotherapist/dramatherapist, not a physician, I have consulted five medical books on epilepsy to get accurate medical information: Epilepsy: a Comprehensive Textbook by Engel and Pedley, Atlas of Epilepsies by Panayiotopoulos and associates (in which I am an associate editor), A Clinical Guide to Epileptic Syndromes and their Treatment by Panayiotopoulos, The Treatment of Epilepsy by Shorvon and associates and Willie's Treatment of Epilepsy: Principles and Practice by Wyllie and associates.

In addition, I sourced information from the most recent literature in medical journals. I have also consulted expert epileptologists.

The book is divided into three parts.

Each chapter of this book is written with the intended reader in mind and supplemented with detailed relevant recommendations for those affected by epilepsy. An abstract at the beginning of each chapter is followed by key words.

The first part (Chaps. 2–15) refers mainly to medical aspects of epilepsy, certain common epileptic syndromes, women and epilepsy, SUDEP (sudden unexpected death in epilepsy), investigations and treatment with emphasis on matters that are helpful for patients to know and appropriate recommendations.

Time limitation on the part of health-care professionals is an important matter that I consider in this book. As I always say: "How much can a doctor do in a thirty minutes medical consultation"? Chapter 3 details recommendations to patients of how to prepare for the medical consultation and take the maximal benefit from it. Prepare well in advance, complete the provided questionnaire, write down what to ask and make sure that you understood well what you were told, what to do and your treatment plan.

In the chapter on women and epilepsy, you will find information and special issues concerning women and particularly those of childbearing age. Potential complications during pregnancy and delivery, risks in drug administration and/or the seizures and potential problems during breastfeeding and childrearing are explained, and quotes of women with epilepsy who live a normal life are presented.

Children with epilepsy and their families are a main concern of this book. Epilepsy in children is extremely diverse from very mild and age limited to severe and progressive. Children with epilepsy, even those with new-onset seizures, are at risk of psychopathology. The whole family may be adversely affected. Parents of children with epilepsy have significant and unmet needs that should be properly addressed from the time of first diagnosis and thus eliminate anxiety and improve quality of life.

Information on adaptations to a different lifestyle from the one they had previously is given to the elderly with epilepsy and their families who have to deal with physical, cognitive and psychosocial changes.

The second part (Chaps. 1 and 16–25) includes the History of Epilepsy, Psychological Treatments and "Metamyth"/Dramatherapy in the treatment of people who have epilepsy, Psychosocial aspects and Stigma in Epilepsy, Complementary, Alternative Treatments, Comorbidities, Safety and Dietary Treatments in epilepsy.

While studying and working in the UK, I was inspired by one of the founders of Dramatherapy and EPR (embodiment, projection, role) theory Sue Jennings and the founder of Role theory Robert Landy from the USA. To make "Metamyth"©, I had the opportunity to share and exchange ideas with both these brilliant tutors who together with others have influenced my work. They are Mary Smail, Jocelyn Quenell, from Sesamy London School of Speech and drama, Dr. Alida Gersey, Brenda Meldrum, Dr. Ditty Dokter, at Anglia Ruskin University Cambridge, Art Therapist Dr Susan Hogan from the School of Health and Sciences at Derby University and Sorel Carson at ALRA (Academy of Live and Recorded Arts) London. Pr. Oliver Taplin from Maugdalen College Oxford and the Archives of Performances of Ancient Greek and Roman Drama and Dr. Moira Davies from the University of the Arts London have also been my guides. In Greece, Dr. Covanis now IBE president has offered me the opportunity to do my research on Parents' reaction and attitude of children with IFE in the child neurology clinic in Agia Sophia Children's Hospital, and the First neurology and psychiatry university clinic in Aeginition Hospital has offered me the opportunity to establish the "Metamyth"© clinic for patients with epilepsy. In the Society of Psychoanalytic group Psychotherapy, Athens, I take a lot of drive and inspiration for my work.

As the founder of "Metamyth"© Psychological Therapy, I devote one chapter to "Metamyth"/Dramatherapy. "Metamyth"© is based on techniques and theories coming from my training as a dramatherapist and developed from research into epilepsy including the psychosocial aspects of this condition. It is influenced by Humanistic, Jungian and Existential Psychotherapies, and it is psychoanalytically oriented.

The patients have been my inspiration in formulating my method. "Metamyth"© can help the patients enjoy life, realize dreams and become significant contributors to society by exploring the archetypal dimensions of the psyche of the person with epilepsy and taking into consideration clinical experience and research.

I devote Chap. 17 to psychogenic nonepileptic seizures, because they are so difficult to distinguish from epileptic seizures. Freud in 1924 writing about Dostoevsky's epilepsy says that it is right to distinguish between an "organic" and an "affective epilepsy". "In the first case the mental life of the patient is subjected to an alien disturbance from without in the second case the disturbance is an expression of his mental life itself".

My research on parental attitude and reactions with children with idiopathic focal epilepsy based on a specifically designed questionnaire and presented in Chap. 24 shows that parents ask for psychological help for themselves and for their children.

The psychological aspects of epilepsy observed since ancient times were misread as demonic and caused people with epilepsy to be persecuted. This created a shadow inherited through the years by people with epilepsy and felt by their families as you will read in Chap. 25 on stigma. The therapist also feels this shadow, and "Metamyth"© is a way to help and heal or dispel it.

The third part details relevant Websites and other current resources for people with epilepsy. Immediate access to proper and accurate information about epilepsy is of great benefit to health-care professionals and patients. People affected by epilepsy often use the wide information provided on the Internet for formulating their own opinion regarding diagnosis and management. I have provided information from the most reliable resources for such information around the world because of a growing concern that a substantial proportion of what is found on the Web might be inaccurate, erroneous, misleading or fraudulent.

An advice I give to patients is: "the more you know the better it is". I say this knowing that some patients do not want to know exactly what is happening to them and this is all right. By cooperating with the doctor, patients can take active part on decisions and on their diagnosis and treatment. Because misdiagnosis is common in epilepsy with approximately one-fifth of patients diagnosed and treated for epilepsy while suffering from other than epilepsy conditions, I provide proper education and information to assist patients in a "shared decision-making" process that allows them to make informed decisions together with their health carers, taking into account the best scientific evidence available in this book as well as their personal values and preferences. In the shared decision-making, patients deserve to be fully informed about their specific health problem and the risks and benefits of treatments, also ensuring that their values and preferences are thoroughly considered.

Although the book is addressed to patients, I believe it will also interest and be useful to physicians, medical students, psychotherapists, psychologists, other health-care professionals, teachers and family of people with epilepsy.

In my book, "The Epilepsy book: A Companion for patients", I put into words my life experience as a therapist and the information, the knowledge, the emotions and the reasoned argument that it holds.

I wish my book to become a good companion to many people and to those who hold it in their hands I wish good reading and enjoyment.

London, UK
May 28, 2017

Thalia Valeta, B.A., M.A., HPC reg.

# Abbreviations

| | |
|---|---|
| ADR | Adverse drug reaction |
| AED | Anti-epileptic drug |
| CNS | Central nervous system |
| ECG | Electrocardiogram |
| EEG | Electroencephalogram |
| FDA | US Food and Drug Administration |
| fMRI | Functional magnetic resonance imaging |
| GTCS | Generalized tonic-clonic seizure |
| IGE | Idiopathic generalized epilepsy |
| IBE | International Bureau for Epilepsy |
| IFE | Idiopathic focal epilepsy |
| ILAE | International League Against Epilepsy |
| JME | Juvenile myoclonic epilepsy |
| MCM | Major congenital malformation |
| MRI | Magnetic resonance imaging |
| SUDEP | Sudden unexpected death in epilepsy |
| WHO | World Health Organization |

**Abstract**

Epilepsy has probably afflicted humans from their early evolution. Epilepsy has been one of the very few diseases that have been associated with so much medical and social attention, debate and misunderstanding. Patients with epilepsy, unlike many persons with other medical diseases, have been unfairly singled-out from medicine, religions and societies, prosecuted, and discriminated as being affected by magic, devils, or supernatural causes. The modern era is marked by significant advances in all aspects of epilepsy.

**Keywords**

Ancient times • Babylonian tablet • Hippocrates • Scientific progress • John Hughlings Jackson • treatment • Modern views

## Ancient Times

The first recorded evidence of epilepsy is found in ancient Indian medicine of the Vedic period of 4500–1500 BC, but the main descriptions of the disease are mainly dated from 2000 BC as documented in the Edwin Smith medical papyrus which was a surgical papyrus from ancient Egypt (1700 BC) and which refers to epileptic convulsions in at least five cases. Descriptions of epilepsy are found also on a Babylonian tablet,(1050 BC) the Indian Ayurvedic literature and the Hippocratic writings in Greece [1–3].

The twenty-fifth tablet of 40 Babylonian cuneiform tablets called Sakkiku (all diseases) dating from 1050 BC is devoted to miqtu (a disease that the person loses consciousness and foams at the mouth) accurately describes many seizure types and their prognosis [3]. A person with a single seizure will live, but if he has two or three seizures a day, he will die. A patient who has a seizure and never regains consciousness will also die. However, the Babylonians believed that supernatural creatures

© Springer International Publishing AG 2017
T. Valeta, *The Epilepsy Book: A Companion for Patients*,
DOI 10.1007/978-3-319-61679-7_1

caused the various manifestations of miqtu, with each seizure type associated with the name of a spirit or god, usually evil. Thus, the demon Lilu, his slave-girl Lili, and his wife Lilitu would possess people, causing their epilepsy. If a person laughs loudly while his limbs are being flexed and extended, it is the hand of Lilu. A curious feature of this family of demons is that they are childless. As a result of their envy, they had a particular interest in possessing children, explaining the frequent occurrence of childhood epilepsy. The Babylonians also had different terms for diurnal and nocturnal epilepsy, and they attributed nocturnal spells to ghosts. They claimed that exclusively nocturnal spells featuring headaches, hissing in the ears, deafness and abdominal distension show the hand of a ghost. Multiple seizures in a single day were attributed to the ghost of a departed murderer, adding that those with this illness will surely die.

In the Indian Ayurvedic literature of Charaka Samhita (which has been dated to 400 BC) epilepsy is described as "apasmara" which means "loss of consciousness". The Charaka Samhita description includes symptomatology, aetiology, diagnosis and treatment of epilepsy.

Real advance in understanding epilepsy was made by Hippocrates (460–370 BC) in ancient Greece who in his famous treatise *"On the sacred disease"* clarified that epilepsy was just a natural disease of the brain and not a sacred one:

*"It is thus with regard to the disease called Sacred: it appears to me to be nowise more divine nor more sacred than other diseases, but has a natural cause from the originates like other affections. Men regard its nature and cause as divine from ignorance and wonder, because it is not at all like to other diseases. And this notion of its divinity is kept up by their inability to comprehend it, and the simplicity of the mode by which it is cured, for men are freed from it by purifications and incantations. But if it is reckoned divine because it is wonderful, instead of one there are many diseases which would be sacred; for, as I will show, there are others no less wonderful and prodigious, which nobody imagines to be sacred."* Hippocrates 400 BC (http://classics.mit.edu/Hippocrates/sacred.html).

Another important contribution was by Galen (131–201 AD) who described aura, three forms of epilepsy and differentiated epilepsy from tetanus.

However, these and subsequently true but scarce scientific views of epilepsy as a natural brain disease have been ignored. In the next 22 centuries and more, patients with epilepsy have been the victims of false ideas, superstition, ignorance, or cruelty from within their own societies, religions, medical and legal institutions, (see Chap. 25 on Stigma).

*"The history of epilepsy can be summarised as 4000 years of ignorance, superstition, and stigma followed by 100 years of knowledge, superstition, and stigma"* Rajendra Kale 1997 [4].

## Medieval Times and Renaissance

In the Medieval times (fifth–fourteenth century) epilepsy was believed to be contagious or mainly the result of demonic possession. (See Chap. 25 on Stigma).

St. Valentine was known for healing people with epilepsy around Europe. The first acknowledgement of St. Valentine being a patron saint for people with epilepsy is printed in The Nuremberg Chronicle, an illustrated book printed in 1493.

The Renaissance (fourteenth–seventeenth century) is marked by an explosion of literature regarding epilepsy. Paracelsus believed that epilepsy has five seats (brain, liver, heart, intestines, limbs), animals can have it and the symptoms can be treated ("prevent the root from growing"). Fernelius supported the theory that poisonous vapors affected the brain and led to epileptic fits, and rejected the belief that epilepsy is contagious. Thomas Willis assumed the existence of a 'spasmodic explosive copula' from the head. Charles Drélincourt provoked epileptic convulsions in a dog by driving a needle into the fourth ventricle of the brain.

Enlightenment flourished in the nineteenth century to the in-depth knowledge achieved to date. However, again the social and legal rights of people with epilepsy have been ruined by brutal acts against them, including legislation schemes in advanced countries in Europe and the USA that prohibited them until recently from marriage and often submitted them to forced sterilization.

## Scientific Progress in the Nineteenth Century

The foundation of our modern understanding of epilepsy was laid in the nineteenth Century with the work of John Hughlings Jackson, a London neurologist, who precisely proposed that seizures were the result of sudden brief electrochemical discharges in the brain. Soon afterwards the electrical excitability of the brain in animals and man was discovered. A major advance was the discovery of human electroencephalography in 1920 by Hans Berger, a German psychiatrist. The EEG has become an indispensable tool in the diagnosis of epilepsy.

## The Modern Era

The modern era is marked by an expansion of interest in basic mechanisms underlying seizures and epilepsies, stimulated by developments in genetics, molecular biology, neurophysiology, functional imaging and numerous neurochemical techniques.

Technological advances have been tremendous in functional and structural brain imaging with significant clinical and research applications. Because of significant advances in neurosurgery this now provides the main effective treatment in many focal epilepsies and mainly mesial temporal lobe epilepsy.

Research in molecular genetics of epilepsy is now in a phase of rapid progress with more than 20 genes and at least some of the important genetic risk factors contributing to epilepsy have been identified. Genetic diagnostic or predictive testing is now available.

## The History of Treatment of Epilepsy

In ancient times, magical, religious diet and medical herbs were the main treatments applied for people with epilepsy. The modern era of pharmacotherapy probably began with bromides (1856), phenobarbital (1912) and phenytoin (1938). In recent decades there has been a proliferation of new antiepileptic drugs (see Chap. 15 on prophylactic drug treatment of epilepsy). Precision treatment of epilepsy is now within our reach. In our days psychological treatments are being used to alleviate the psychological comorbidities of epilepsy (see Chap. 16, 17 and 18). Metamyth" © (Chap. 19) is an innovative approach in psychotherapy for people with epilepsy.

## Psychosocial Advances

During the last few decades greater attention has been paid to quality of life and psychosocial issues, for people with epilepsy, although progress is slow and services are still poor in most parts of the world [5]. In 1997 the International League Against Epilepsy and the International Bureau for Epilepsy joined forces with the World Health Organization to establish the Global Campaign Against Epilepsy to address these issues [6]. The aim of this Global Campaign is to improve prevention, treatment, care and services for people with epilepsy. It also aims to raise public awareness about the disorder. The legal social and work rights of people with epilepsy are now largely recognized.

"Humanity must now remember what history has taught us and take responsibility to create new foundations in the way epilepsy is understood in the present, so that change takes place and history does not repeat its dark pages. Instead, create an opportunity to see people who have epilepsy on the basis of their abilities". Thalia Valeta 2010 [7].

## Recommended Readings

- Atlas Epilepsy Care in the World, World Health Organization: http://www.who.int/mental_health/neurology/Epilepsy_atlas_r1.pdf
- Epilepsy Museum Kork: http://www.epilepsiemuseum.de/english/
- Highlights in the history of epilepsy: https://www.hindawi.com/journals/ert/2014/582039/ And http://cdn.intechopen.com/pdfs/21744.pdf
- History of the treatment of epilepsy: http://www.epilepsiemuseum.de/alt/body_therapieen.html
- Sociocultural history of epilepsy: http://www.epilepsiestiftung-wolf.de/resources/10+Sociocultural+history.pdf
- History of epilepsy timeline: https://epilepsyed.org/history-of-epilepsy/
- Hippocrates 400 BC: http://classics.mit.edu/Hippocrates/sacred.html

## References

1. Bladin PF, Eadie MJ. Medical aspects of the history of epilepsy. In: Panayiotopoulos CP, editor and Valeta T, section editor. Atlas of epilepsies. London: Springer; 2010; p. 27–33.
2. Temkin O. The falling sickness: a history of epilepsy from the greeks to the beginnings of modern neurology. Baltimore: Johns Hopkins University Press; 1994.
3. Magiorkinis E, Sidiropoulou K, Diamantis A. Hallmarks in the history of epilepsy: epilepsy in antiquity. Epilepsy Behav. 2010;17:103–8.
4. Kale R. Bringing epilepsy out of the shadows. BMJ. 1997;315:2–3.
5. Wolf P. Sociocultural history of epilepsy. In: Panayiotopoulos CP, editor and Valeta T, section editor. Atlas of epilepsies London: Springer; 2010; p. 35–43.
6. World Health Organization. Atlas epilepsy care in the world 2005. Geneva: World Health Organisation; 2005.
7. Valeta T. Historical aspects of epilepsy: overview. In: Panayiotopoulos CP, editor and Valeta T, section editor. Atlas of epilepsies. London:Springer; 2010; p. 25–26.

# General Aspects of Epilepsy

**2**

**Abstract**

"Epilepsy" refers to many brain diseases having in common the occurrence of epileptic seizures. Patients with epilepsy show significant differences in severity, types, manifestations and causes of epileptic seizures, management, coexisting illnesses, and varying psychosocial, educational and employment impacts on individuals and their families.

**Keywords**

Epilepsy • Seizures • Prevalence • Cause • Diagnosis • Treatment • Outcome

## What is Epilepsy?

Epilepsy is a brain disease defined by recurrent (repeated), unprovoked seizures which are often unpredictable. Epilepsy is a spectrum condition with a wide range of seizure types and control varying from person-to-person.

"Epilepsy" is not a single disease or a single abnormal condition but symptoms of numerous and often different disorders having in common the occurrence of epileptic seizures. In other words, epilepsy is a variety of disorders with significant differences in their severity, types and manifestations of seizures and causes, coexisting illnesses, and varying psychosocial, educational and employment impacts on individuals and their families. The use of plural "epilepsies" is in order to emphasise their immense diversities in manifestations, cause, management and prognosis.

The epilepsies

- may be mild or severe
- occur in a certain period of life only or be life long
- seizures may be the only clinical manifestation but others may be associated with variable fixed or progressive physical and mental symptoms

- may be caused by variable brain lesions (injuries, stroke, tumours) or a genetic/hereditary predisposition to seizures
- may respond well or be resistant to treatment
- may impose little or severe handicap in the life of the patient and the family.

Some patients may not require antiepileptic drug treatments while in others therapy may be lifelong.

## What are the Formal Scientific Definitions of Epilepsy

The International League against Epilepsy (ILAE) has a conceptual and a practical definition of epilepsy.

The conceptual ILAE definition is [1]:

Epilepsy is a disorder of the brain characterised by an enduring predisposition to generate epileptic seizures and by the neurobiological, cognitive, psychological and social consequences of this condition. This definition of epilepsy 'requires the occurrence of at least one epileptic seizure' with the precondition that this is 'in association with an enduring disturbance of the brain capable of giving rise to other seizures' [1].

The operational (practical) ILAE definition of epilepsy is: [2].

Epilepsy is a disease of the brain defined by any of the following conditions

1. At least two unprovoked (or reflex) seizures occurring >24 hours apart
2. One unprovoked (or reflex) seizure and a probability of further seizures similar to the general recurrence risk (at least 60%) after two unprovoked seizures, occurring over the next 10 years
3. Diagnosis of an epilepsy syndrome

## What is the Difference Between Epileptic Seizures and Epilepsy?

Epileptic seizures are a symptom of epilepsy. Having a single seizure does not necessarily mean that a person has epilepsy. People with seizures provoked only by fever or alcohol-withdrawal or acute head injury are not diagnosed as having epilepsy, because these people do not have epileptic seizures in the absence of such factors.

Many people with epilepsy have more than one type of seizure and may have other symptoms of neurological problems as well.

An epileptic seizure is a short event of symptoms which are caused by a burst of abnormal electrical activity in the brain. This causes different symptoms, depending on the location of the electrical burst (discharge), how it spreads and how long it lasts. Some seizures are very mild and can hardly be noticed, while others are totally disabling. The duration of epileptic seizures is usually brief for seconds to 3–4 min and then they stop spontaneously.

For details see Chap. 4 on epileptic seizures.

## How Common is Epilepsy?

Epilepsy is a common brain disorder that affects all ages and all races of both sexes. Epileptic seizures affect 1–2% of the population and this is higher amongst children. In developed countries, 6–7% of children will suffer at least one or more epileptic seizures (provoked or unprovoked) and this is probably double in resource-poor countries (7–15% of children).

In developed countries each year 50 out of 100,000 people will develop epilepsy and active epilepsy (people with epilepsy at any given point in time) is between 4 and 7 per 1000 people. An apparent decline of the incidence of epilepsy in recent studies may be attributed to better diagnosis, improved prenatal care and decreased exposure of children to risk factors, such as severe head trauma and nervous system infections.

## Cause, Diagnosis, Treatment and Outcome of Epilepsy

### What is the Cause of Epilepsy?

Any brain disorder that disturbs the structure or the function of the brain can cause epilepsy. These include birth defects, brain tumours, infections, injuries, ischemia or anoxia, cerebrovascular disease, malformations of cortical development, chromosomal abnormalities, neurocutaneous disorders, degenerative brain disorders. Some epilepsies are genetically determined; that means that certain genes can cause brain disorders that manifest with epileptic seizures alone or with other physical and mental symptoms.

The cause of epilepsy cannot be documented in approximately half of all people with epilepsy. This is sometimes called "idiopathic epilepsy"—which just means that we don't know the cause of it. Some people have a naturally low resistance to having seizures (a low 'seizure threshold') which can be in their genetic make-up.

### What is Epileptic Syndrome?

An epileptic syndrome is an epileptic disorder characterised by a cluster of signs and symptoms customarily occurring together; these include such items as the type of seizure, aetiology, anatomy, precipitating factors, age of onset, severity, chronicity, diurnal and circadian cycling, and sometimes prognosis.

See details in Chap. 7 on epileptic syndromes.

### How Epilepsy is Diagnosed?

The diagnosis of epilepsy is almost always based solely on the clinical history obtained from the patient and witnesses. Electroencephalography (EEG) and brain imaging are the main diagnostic procedures. See Chap. 14.

## How Epilepsy is Treated?

The aim of therapy in epilepsy is:

- total freedom or maximal reduction of seizures and particularly the severe ones
- no significant side effects from drugs
- best quality of life with regard to physical, mental, educational, social and psychological functioning of the patient

The main treatment is usually with antiepileptic drugs (antiseizure drugs) (AEDs) taken daily for as long as the patient has active epilepsy. With a properly selected single AED (monotherapy), 50–70% of patients achieve seizure freedom. Combination of more than one AED (polytherapy) should be avoided if possible, but it is needed for about 30–50% of patients whose seizures are not controlled with one drug. However, AEDs are ineffective for about 20% of patients. These patients are candidates for neurosurgical interventions, other pharmacological or non-pharmacological treatments.

A precondition for any treatment is that the patient truly suffers epileptic seizures. Correct seizure and often syndrome diagnosis is a must for the success of therapeutic decisions because the choice of AED primarily depends on seizure type, whereas length of treatment is mainly determined by syndrome type.

See details in Chap. 15 prophylactic treatment of epilepsy.

## What is the Outcome (Prognosis) of Epilepsy?

Epileptic seizures, particularly if convulsive, are serious paroxysmal events with significant psychosocial impact and in children they may affect cognition and behaviour. Serious injuries may occur as a result of seizures. The prognosis of epilepsy is dramatically diverse according to aetiology and epileptic syndrome. Overall, nearly half of patients with newly diagnosed epilepsy enter long and sustained remission. Idiopathic/genetic epilepsy (i.e. without documented lesions in the brain) is more likely to remit or be controlled with AED than symptomatic/structural epilepsy (i.e. with structural lesions in the brain). Certain types of idiopathic childhood epilepsy resolve or improve with age. Conversely, certain types of symptomatic epilepsy are life long, intractable or relentlessly progressive. Many patients have additional psychiatric, behavioural, neurological and intellectual disturbances. Depression, suicidal and mortality risk is at least two to three times higher in patients with epilepsy than in the general population [3]. Support is needed through psychological family management. (See Chap. 18 on Psychological treatments for epilepsy). Many people with epilepsy have lived with this condition and have distinguished themselves in various disciplines.

Epilepsy is considered to be resolved for individuals who had an age-dependent epilepsy syndrome (self-limited) but are now past the applicable age or those who have remained seizure-free for the last 10 years, with no medication for the last 5 years [2].

## Recommendations for Patients with Epilepsy and Their Family

If you or your child is diagnosed as having epilepsy or epileptic seizures, the first and more important legitimate question to ask is what type of epilepsy and what type of epileptic seizures.

This then defines other important matters that you should know such as whether prophylactic medication is needed, what is the optional antiepileptic drug to use, length of treatment, prognosis, safety measures, educational and social consequences.

The information you find in this chapter will help you in a good collaboration and partnership with the treating physician to reach a successful outcome.

Parents and patients often use the wide information provided on the internet to formulate their own opinion about diagnosis and management. They are entitled and should be encouraged to do so, in order to develop their awareness and communication as part of their partnership with their healthcare professionals. In the last section of this book Chap. 26 I provide information about reliable websites and other resources like books, formal guidelines and practice parameters for people with epilepsy.

## Recommended Readings

- http://www.ilae.org/commission/class/diagnostic.cfm
  This is the ILAE EpilepsyDiagnosis.org which an excellent online diagnostic manual of the epilepsies which provides information of how to diagnose seizure type(s), classify epilepsy, diagnose epilepsy syndromes and define the aetiology.
- https://www.epilepsy.org.uk/info/syndromes
  This is a detail guideline and support for patients with epilepsy in the Epilepsy Action which is the UK's leading epilepsy organisation.
- http://www.epilepsy.com/learn/types-epilepsy-syndromes
  http://www.epilepsy.com/information/professionals/about-epilepsy-seizures/overview-epilepsy-syndromes
  This is a detail guideline and support for patients with epilepsy in The Epilepsy Foundation of the USA and epilepsy.com.
- https://www.epilepsysociety.org.uk/what-epilepsy#.WE7PhPmLTIU
  This is a very useful website about epilepsy of the British Epilepsy Society.
- http://www.ncbi.nlm.nih.gov/books/NBK2606/

## References

1. Fisher RS, van Emde BW, Blume W, Elger C, Genton P, Lee P, et al. Epileptic seizures and epilepsy: definitions proposed by the International League Against Epilepsy (ILAE) and the International Bureau for Epilepsy (IBE). Epilepsia. 2005;46:470–2.

2. Fisher RS, Acevedo C, Arzimanoglou A, Bogacz A, Cross JH, Elger CE, et al. ILAE Official Report: a practical clinical definition of epilepsy. Epilepsia. 2014;55:475–82.
3. Valeta T. Impact of newly identified epileptic seizures in patients and family. In: Panayiotopoulos CP, editor. Newly identified epileptic seizures: diagnosis, procedures and management, vol. 3. Oxford: Medicinae; 2007. p. 138–44.

# Preparing for the Medical Consultation

3

**Abstract**

The medical consultation is the main opportunity for the doctor to explore the patient's problems, make the correct diagnosis and provide the appropriate management. This chapter details recommendations to patients of how to prepare for the medical consultation and take the maximal benefit from it. Prepare well in advance, complete the provided questionnaire and be aware of time limitations.

**Keywords**

Medical consultation • Epilepsy • History • Questionnaire • Recommendations

## What is the Significance of Appropriate Preparation of the Medical Consultation?

The medical consultation is the main opportunity for the doctor to explore the patient's problems and concerns and to start to identify the reasons for their ill health.

Obtaining all the relevant information is crucial in helping your physician to formulate a correct diagnosis, request the proper tests and possibly prescribe medication.

One way to make the most out of your appointment with your physician is to prepare in advance as much as possible.

## Providing an Accurate History Is Vital to a Correct Diagnosis

A correct diagnosis starts with gathering a history (information) about the event/s that is of concern to you. Your physician needs to have a full picture of your health and not just of epilepsy. Your lifestyle, habits, alcohol consumption, recreational

© Springer International Publishing AG 2017
T. Valeta, *The Epilepsy Book: A Companion for Patients*,
DOI 10.1007/978-3-319-61679-7_3

drugs, sleep patterns, emotional stress, any past surgeries, injuries, or medical problems and any special concerns are important to disclose and discuss.

**Write Down**
(a)  your medical history (see samples below)
(b)  your list of questions (consider the time limitations)

**Bring with you**
(a)  all your important medical records such as notes from other doctors, seizure calendars, lab results.
(b)  list of any medications, vitamins, dietary supplements, or herbal treatments you are taking or have taken in the past and particularly around the time that the events have happened to you

It is advisable and of help if you have a friend or relative present during your consultation. These have to know you well, dedicated to you, intelligent and understand that their role is to help you and your physician without unnecessary destructions.

## Attending for a Probable First Seizure

If you attend for a first seizure you should use the following guidance of what is usually requested in your first attendance. I use the term event because what happened to you may not be an epileptic seizure and there are many examples of misdiagnosis.

## History of the Event

Name:____ Date of birth:_____.
Address:

### Description and Sequence of the Event
How this started and how this progressed.
   *Important aspects to describe are whether you lost consciousness (gradually or suddenly?), whether you had convulsions (whole body and limbs? one or both sides?) and for how long.
   During this event and before recovery (a) were you pale or blue (b) sweating or dry (c) salivate (d) eyes were open or closed? Urine and/or faeces incontinent? Tongue biting?
   After the event were you back to your Normal? Confused? Had headache? Cried? And for how long?
   Did you obtain any injuries?

### Date and Approximate Time That This Happened
Early morning after awakening? Any other time of the day? In sleep?

## Place and Circumstances at the Time of the Incidence

At home? Work? Restaurant? Pub? Disco? Standing, sitting or lying down. Awake or asleep.

## Precipitating Factors

There are many factors that can precipitate seizures and these include: flickering lights, alcohol consumption, sleep deprivation, tiredness, stress, hunger, thirst, physical illness, fever. Certain medicines and recreational substances may also induce seizures and these should be discussed with your physician.

For women: menstrual cycle or pregnancy should be included in the discussion of possible precipitating factors.

## Witnesses

It is important to substantiate your description with that of witnesses. Having their own written accounts of the events is often crucial.

Attending health professionals/ambulance/accident and emergency of hospital (name and address if known).

Results of relevant tests and copies of letters if you attended other health care facilities.

## Symptoms and Warnings Prior to Losing Consciousness (If This Happened)

These are sometimes difficult to describe and may include: "stomach sensation (pain, strange feeling) ascending towards my neck", "strange sensation as if I had not being in this place before", "not recognising familiar persons who were with me", "dizziness and faint sensations", "visual or hearing disturbances", "numbness in the left/right of my face, hand, leg", "jerking of my eyelids, hands, legs". Their duration?

In all these occasions try to be as descriptive as possible with your own words.

Did any of these symptoms happen to you before the major event and in other occasions? If Yes, provide details.

## Personal and Family History

It is also important to have in writing a brief account of your personal and family history.

Personal history: Born and developed well?, significant illnesses and/or brain injuries, febrile seizures or other epileptic events in the past.

Family history: Epileptic seizures and/or other illnesses in parents, siblings and close relatives.

## Attending for Recurrent (Repeated) Seizures

If you attend for recurrent epileptic seizures for which you have a diagnosis of "epilepsy" you should use the following questionnaire which is based on a previously validated questionnaire [1].

Your neurologist needs to know about your past seizures to help predict the course of your epilepsy. To help inform your neurologist of past and current seizure activity, keep track of the details and circumstances surrounding your seizures in a seizure diary.

## Questionnaire to Complete for Patients with Recurrent Seizures

Name:____ Date of birth:_____.
Address:

**Give a brief history of your seizures**
Previous hospitals and physicians you have seen for your epileptic seizures (please write in order with dates and addresses if possible).
Results of previous tests (particularly EEG and brain MRI or CT scan).
Were your seizures ever recorded with video? (This is usually very helpful particularly for patients who have frequent seizures).
Other medical conditions?
Psychological disturbances?
Social effects?

**Do you have One or different types of the following list of seizures?**
(a) Generalised convulsions with loss of consciousness that always come out of the blue without any warning?
(b) Generalised convulsions with loss of consciousness that always follow other symptoms/warnings?
(c) Focal seizures consisting of various sensations and/or one sided convulsions without losing consciousness
(d) Focal seizures consisting of various sensations and/or one sided convulsions which may progress to loss of consciousness
(e) Focal seizures consisting of various sensations and/or one sided convulsions with loss of consciousness from the beginning
(f) Absence seizures (blank spells or spells in which you "switch off or go into a trance?"
(g) Jerks (muscle twitches that may make you drop things or fall?) especially just after waking up. Please be aware that jerks which happen as you go to sleep are normal phenomena.

**For each seizure type please describe**
1. what happens in each type of seizure?
2. how frequently do you have each type of seizure?
3. at what age did each type of seizure started?
4. at what age did each type of seizure stopped?
5. at what age each type of seizure was more severe and more frequent

**Do you have any warning before seizures occur? Describe the warning**
- How long does the warning last?
- Does the warning ever occur on its own?

**Do you "go blank" or lose consciousness of your surroundings during the seizure?**
- For how long does this last?
- Are you completely blank (and unresponsive) or retain some awareness and responsiveness (answering for example with yes or no to questions)
- Do you stop what you are doing or continue on automatically "like a robot?"

**If you do not lose consciousness**
- Do your legs give way?
- Do you drop to ground?
- Do your arms and/or head drop?
- Do you drop objects?
- Do you become emotional and cry? (describe it)

**During a seizure do you experience any of the following (describe it in your own words and give duration)**
- a feeling of being in a dream or in an unusually strange or familiar place?
- intense fear? rage or anger? euphoria, happiness, or pleasure?
- flashbacks or memories of past events (as though you are reliving the past)?
- the sense that everyday surroundings or objects are unfamiliar?
- seeing or hearing things that are not real?
- unusual smells or tastes?
- pins and needles, electric shocks, tingling, or other changes in sensation? (Where does the change in sensation start and how does it spread?)
- objects or sounds in your environment appearing distorted or altered?
- a feeling that everything is in slow motion or speed up?
- a funny feeling in your stomach?
- mouth watering or drooling?
- palpitations or a pounding heart?
- sweating
- eyes flickering
- movements or jerks of any particularly part of your face, limbs

**During a seizure were you told by witnesses that any of the following symptoms occur? (describe them and give duration)**
- Eyes closed or open, rolling upwards or turning in a particular direction (At what stage of the seizure? Which direction do they turn? And for how long)
- The head turn in a particular direction?
- The arms are jerking or rigid? bent or straight? in what position? One or both arms?

- The legs are jerking or rigid? bent or straight? in what position? One or both legs?
- Breathing normal? Stops? Difficult? (At what stage of the seizure? For how long)
- If convulsing and jerking, are the jerks infrequent and irregular, or are they repeated and regular?
- Smacking of the lips, licking of the lips, chewing, swallowing, laughing, picking at or fiddling with things, walking or making stepping or bicycling movements, speaking?

**During a seizure**
- Do you ever bite your tongue (which side?)
- Do you wet yourself (at what stage? Beginning or end?)

**After a seizure**
- are you confused or drowsy? Describe how you feel and duration
- do you have a headache (one side or both?). Describe it.
- vomit and other effects?
- any effects on vision, speech, sensation, or muscle power? Describe the changes.

**Do your seizures follow a particular pattern/sequence? Describe the pattern**

**Do you think that any seizure type**
- occurs predominately during any particular time of the day or in sleep?
- occurs in relation to any particular date of your menstrual cycle?
- is precipitated by particular factor/s? sleep deprivation, emotional stress, excessive alcohol, flickering lights, fever, closing of the eyes, bright lights, TV, video games, discos, reading, mental concentration, excitement?

**Are you on any medication?**
- If yes, which drugs?
- How long have you been taking this medication?
- Were you on any other medication before?
- Do you think any particular drug helped you more?
- Do you think any particular drug made you worse (increased the frequency of any type of seizure or significant side effects?

**Family history**
- Are you aware of any other member of your family (first and second-degree relatives) having epilepsy? Provide as many details as you know for each of the affected members of your family.

## Provide a Diary of Your Seizures

You may make a diary yourself by noting the date and time of your seizures. Alternatively you can use seizure diaries you can find in the internet or in the epilepsy clinic you attend. PLEASE, ADD HERE ANYTHING ELSE YOU MAY FEEL THAT IT IS RELEVANT.

## While You Are with Your Physician

Make sure that your physician has read the information that you have forwarded to him/her prior to your appointment. It is likely that you have to go step by step with him/her.

Your physician is likely to ask more details and emphasise on:

- The symptoms you experience and those observed by witnesses
- Sensations and other symptoms just before the onset of a convulsive event
- Frequency, timing and severity of the seizures
- When did the seizures started and under what circumstances
- Triggers and precipitating factors
- What, if anything, seems to improve your seizures?
- What, if anything, appears to worsen your seizures?

Your friend or relative may make notes during the consultation so you can recall later the advice provided. If you are unsure about something or do not understand the language being used, the best time to ask for clarification is during the appointment.

If medicines are prescribed, the course of treatment and possible side effects should also be discussed. Do not forget that your physician provides you with recommendations for your informed decisions particularly when referring to medications.

## At the End of Your Consultation

Try to have a clear understanding of what you were told, what to do and your treatment plan. Ask for written instructions. Make sure that you have some answers to your questions such as:

- how to take medications
- know what to do if another seizure occurs or if you miss your medication
- Is this an epileptic seizure/epilepsy? If yes, what is the likely cause of it?
- Is this a one off event or recurrent?
- If recurrent, what type of epilepsy is this?
- What kind of tests do I need?
- What safety measures I have to follow for myself and others if I have another seizure?
- Are there any restrictions that I need to follow?

There are of course so many other questions particularly of specific groups of patients like women of child bearing age, pregnant or caring for a baby.

## Recommendations for Patients with Epilepsy and Their Family

Due to time constraints of a medical consultation not all aspects of your health may be dealt with and some of your questions may not be answered or details are missing [2]. Most of these matters can be explained to you in the clinic by other health professionals specialising in epilepsy such as nurses, psychologists and counsellors, social workers, pharmacists. I will encourage you not to hesitate to ask for an appointment with a psychologist psychotherapist if you think you need to discuss any issues. You can also educate yourself through reading books, (this one for example is a companion for the patients) educational pamphlets, and dedicated websites for epilepsy. (see resources in Chap. 26 and recommendations and websites for details and further reading at the end of each chapter of this book).

You also have to remember that the advice you read often refers to "epilepsy" in general which may not be appropriate or relevant to the particular type of epilepsy that you have. See Chaps. 7–12 in this book.

My suggestion is to start your self-education by understanding well your own type of epilepsy which determines prognosis, management, avoidance of precipitating factors, likely timing of seizures, and cause. See epileptic syndromes, Chap. 7.

This may sound as a lot of work to do but it is worth it considering that such an effort may contribute to the appropriate diagnosis and management and the importance that these may make in your or your child's life.

In conclusion:

- Be well prepared for the medical consultation and have your information and questions in writing.
- The diagnosis of an epileptic seizure is mainly based on the clinical history, subjective and objective symptoms, witness statements and if possible video recorded events
- A physician usually has limited time (30–45 min) to gather all the information needed for accurate diagnosis, aetiology and prescribing tests needed and possible treatment. Time management is important when preparing for the consultation. Ideally you should aim to avoid appearing rushed, and ensure that you set aside adequate time. Time constraints are often outside a clinician's immediate control and one has to be pragmatic and comply with clinic appointment times.
- A medical interview can be a stressful situation; significant information may be forgotten or missed and important questions may not be asked.
- If you are fully prepared for your consultation you will receive the greatest benefit from your appointment. For example, preparing notes and a list of the questions you want to ask is useful. If the nurse or doctor believes a prescription is necessary they will also need to know the details of any other prescription or over-the-counter medicines that you are taking.

## Recommended Readings

- NICE (National Institute for Health and Care Excellence). Epilepsies: diagnosis and management. http://www.nice.org.uk/guidance/cg137
- NCBI (The National Center for Biotechnology Information Bookshelf). The Epilepsies: Seizures, syndromes and management. http://www.ncbi.nlm.nih.gov/books/NBK2606/

## References

1. Reutens DC, Howell RA, Gebert KE, Berkovic SF. Validation of a questionnaire for clinical seizure diagnosis. Epilepsia. 1992;33:1065–71.
2. Cunningham C, Newton R, Appleton R, Hosking G, McKinlay I. Epilepsy—giving the diagnosis. A survey of British paediatric neurologists. Seizure. 2002;11:500–11.

# Epileptic Seizures

**4**

**Abstract**

Epileptic seizures are short-lived events of symptoms caused by bursts of abnormal electrical activity in the brain. The symptoms depend on the brain areas affected by the electrical discharges. Epileptic seizures are generalized or focal. It is important to know what type of seizures you have because often the treatment differs from one to another type. It is also significant to recognize the symptoms of minor epileptic seizures because these define the affected area of the brain and may warn you on a forthcoming major convulsive seizure.

**Keywords**

Seizures • Epilepsy • Generalized convulsions • Absence seizures • Myoclonic seizures • Focal aware seizures • Focal impaired awareness seizures • Reflex seizures

## What Is an Epileptic Seizure?

An epileptic seizure is scientifically defined as "a transient occurrence of signs and/ or symptoms due to abnormal excessive or synchronous neuronal activity in the brain" [1]. In other words, an epileptic seizure is a short event of symptoms which is caused by a burst of abnormal electrical activity in the brain.

The brain is made up of around 80 billion of specialised nerve cells all of which are interconnected and communicate by constantly sending and receiving tiny electrical impulses/messages. The brain is responsible for all the functions of our mind and body. In a brain which is working normally these functions are well balanced and work together, starting and stopping messages as need arises. An epileptic seizure happens when there is an abnormal and sudden burst of intense electrical activity which causes a temporary disruption to the way the brain normally works. This causes different symptoms, depending on the location of the electrical burst (discharge) and how it spreads. Typically, a seizure lasts from a few seconds to a few minutes.

In the long chapter that follows I present an account of the many types of seizures.

## What Are the Symptoms of Epileptic Seizures?

Symptoms of epileptic seizures may be

- subjective (perceived by the patient only),
- objective (witnessed by observers), or
- both [1].

They include convulsions, abnormal movements, changes of consciousness, memory, sensation, behaviour or functions of the autonomic nervous system.

Major convulsive seizures are the worse and raise personal concerns and draw medical attention because of their dramatic features the consequences on the health and the effect they have on patients and their family. Minor seizures such as absences, mild myoclonic jerks, subjective internal sensations such as auras, psychic or mental symptoms are likely to be unnoticed until they are diagnosed and treated.

## What Are the Types of Epileptic Seizure?

There are many different types of epileptic seizure, and how a seizure affects one person might be different from how it affects someone else. Specific epileptic seizure types are defined by their clinical symptoms and electric (electroencephalographic) manifestations (electroclinical features).

The epileptic seizures are grossly grouped into two major classes: [2–6]

1. *focal or partial epileptic seizures* which originate from a localised brain area (focus) and
2. *generalized epileptic seizures* which affect the whole brain simultaneously
3. *unclassified epileptic seizures* which cannot be confidently diagnosed as either focal or generalized.

## Focal Epileptic Seizures

About 60% of people with epilepsy have focal (partial) seizures. These seizures can often be mild or unusual, and may go unnoticed or be mistaken for anything from intoxication to daydreaming.

The scientific definition is "Focal epileptic seizures are conceptualized as originating within networks limited to one hemisphere. They may be discretely localized or more widely distributed" [4].

**Fig. 4.1** The hemisphere of the brain and its lobes

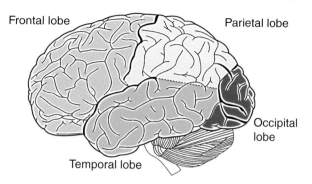

Focal seizures start in one area of the brain (called epileptic focus) and may spread to other regions of the brain. It might affect a large part of one hemisphere or just a small area in one of the lobes. The symptoms of focal seizures depend on the specific area of the brain and what that part of the brain normally does (Fig. 4.1) [2–4].

The brain has two sides called hemispheres. The cerebral hemispheres consist of four lobes which have functional differences. The symptoms of focal seizures depend on which part of the brain is being affected by seizure activity.

**Temporal lobe seizures:** When the seizure activity starts in the temporal lobe the person has symptoms of: ascending (rising) abdominal (epigastric) aura and fear, experiential and complex internal sensations and illusions, auditory, olfactory and gustatory hallucinations, vestibular phenomena, language disturbances and automatisms.

Ascending epigastric sensation of discomfort in the stomach is probably the most characteristic feature of this type of epileptic seizure. Irrespective of how it feels (strange, pressure, pain-like), this sensation often moves upwards in a slow or fast fashion (within seconds) and, interestingly, it is when it reaches the level of the throat that the patient loses consciousness.

Fear is the second commonest aura in temporal lobe seizures: "I am scared, I am in a terrible panic".

Experiential and complex internal sensations and illusions include déjà vu which is a false feeling of having experienced, seen and heard something before as happening now. Please note that déjà vu is experienced by most normal people and the term is used in everyday life. Its significance in epilepsy is when it is present and related with other symptoms and sequence of other epileptic events that may precede, coincide or follow it.

Automatisms are well coordinated movements which occur out of time and space while the patient is unaware of them. These include: simple gestures, such as finger rubbing, lip smacking, chewing, or swallowing, or more complex actions, such as walking away, eating without food.

**Frontal lobe seizures:** When the seizure activity starts in the frontal lobe: the person has localised motor manifestations (stiffness, twitching of tonic, clonic, postural or hypermotor seizures) and complex gestural automatisms. Jerking of the corner of the mouth and thumb is typical of frontal lobe seizures. Hypermotor seizures consist of bizarre, sudden and explosive, bilateral and asymmetric movements and posturing of limbs and body often with strange sounds. They usually occur in sleep.

**Parietal lobe seizures:** When the seizure activity starts in the parietal lobe the person feels numbness or tingling (somatosensory symptoms) localised in one part of the face, arms or legs, disturbances of body image (somatic illusions of an arm or leg bigger or smaller than it actually is), vertiginous, visual illusions, or formed visual hallucinations.

**Occipital lobe seizures:** When the seizure activity starts in the occipital lobe the person experiences visual hallucinations of coloured or flashing lights or seeing something that it is not actually there, visual illusions and oculomotor symptoms.

**Focal epileptic seizures are also subdivided in:**
*Simple focal seizures or focal aware seizures and*
*Complex focal seizures or focal impaired awareness seizures*

**In simple focal seizures, t**he patient is aware of them, remains alert and recalls the events. Aura is a type of simple focal seizure, experienced as a subjective sensation that sometimes act as a warning for an approaching generalized or complex focal seizure. During a simple focal seizure, the patient may experience muscular jerks or strange sensations in one arm or leg, feel, hear, see, smell, or taste odd sensations. Symptoms of a simple focal seizure include:

- changes in the way things look, smell, feel, taste or sound
- an intense feeling that events have happened before (déjà vu)
- tingling sensations, or 'pins and needles', in your arms and legs
- sudden intense emotion, such as fear or joy
- twitches or spasms (stiffness) localized in one part of the face, arms, legs

There is no loss of awareness. A simple focal seizure usually lasts just a few seconds or minutes. For each individual these seizures are stereotypical that is the same movement or sensation tends to recur each time a seizure occurs. It is often difficult for patients to describe their symptoms of simple focal seizures. During the seizure they may feel 'strange' but not able to describe the feeling.

**In complex focal seizures**, the patient is unaware of them (loss of consciousness), confused and partly or totally unresponsive. Patients may stare blankly and usually make meaningless repetitive movements which are called automatisms. These include lip smacking, picking at cloths, utter meaningless words, walk around or perform uninhibited actions. During complex focal seizures, patients are not aware of these events, actions and surroundings, or of what they are doing. This type of seizure can arise from any part of the brain but most commonly arises from bilateral involvement of the temporal lobe.

After a complex focal seizure, the person may be confused for a while, sometimes called 'post-ictal' (after seizure) confusion. It may be hard to tell when the seizure has ended. The person might be tired and want to rest. They may not remember the seizure afterwards.

Note: The recent ILAE Commission on classification renames the simple focal epileptic seizures as focal aware seizures and the complex focal seizures as focal impaired awareness seizures. See http://onlinelibrary.wiley.com/doi/10.1111/pi.13670/full

Any type of focal seizure may spread in other parts of the brain and progress to more serious manifestations and convulsions which are called secondarily or generalized tonic clonic seizures of focal onset.

## Generalized Epileptic Seizures

In generalized epileptic seizures the abnormal electrical epileptogenic discharge simultaneously affect both brain hemispheres from onset to termination.

The scientific definition is: "Generalized epileptic seizures are conceptualized as originating at some point within, and rapidly engaging, bilaterally distributed networks. Such bilateral networks can include cortical and subcortical structures, but do not necessarily include the entire cortex" [4].

Generalized seizures may be convulsive or non-convulsive and their main types are:

- Generalized tonic clonic seizures
- Absence seizures
- Myoclonic seizures
- Tonic seizures
- Atonic seizures

**Generalized tonic-clonic seizures (GTCS)** are the most dramatic and serious type. GTCS manifest with sudden loss of consciousness, generalized convulsions and autonomic disturbances. The patient suddenly falls on the ground unconscious and convulsing for 2–3 min. The convulsions are first tonic (all muscles become rigid) and then clonic (repetitive and brief contractions-relaxations of muscles). Autonomic disturbances include cessation of breathing, hypertension, and often incontinence. Recovery is usually slow and the patient remains confused, tired and sleepy 10–30 min or longer after the end of the GTCS. Many patients sustain injuries or burns during a GTCS. Significant points to remember is that the eyes are open during the convulsions and incontinence of urine (when this happens) it occurs only in the immediate postictal phase.

GTCS may have a focal onset (secondarily generalized tonic clonic seizures or focal onset tonic clonic seizures) in which case they are preceded or develop in the course of a focal epileptic seizure.

**Absence seizures** consist of a brief for a few seconds loss of consciousness which is abrupt at onset and termination. The patient stops what is doing and may have a blank stare with possibly a brief upward rotation of the eyes. If the patient is speaking, speech is slowed or interrupted; if walking, he stands transfixed; if eating, the food will stop on his way to the mouth. Usually the patient will be unresponsive when spoken to. In some, attacks are aborted when the patient is spoken to. The attack lasts from a few seconds to half a minute and terminates as rapidly as it started. Absence seizures, usually severe and frequent, mainly occur in children. In adults they are milder and less frequent.

The absence seizures are fundamentally different from other types of seizure, which also makes their treatment different.

Please, also note that absence seizures are often confused with complex focal seizures which is a significant error because the treatment, cause and prognosis are different.

**Myoclonic jerks** are brief for a few seconds sudden, shock-like movements/ twitches of limb muscles or the body that may result in falls. Most normal people experience myoclonic jerks as they are drifting to sleep (hypnagogic jerks) which are entirely normal phenomena.

**Generalized tonic seizures** are convulsive attacks of sustained muscular contractions only (stiffness, rigidity of the muscles), without clonic components. They usually last a few seconds but sometimes minutes. They may be numerous during sleep. They mainly occur in severe forms of epilepsy such as Lennox-Gastaut syndrome and they often cause forceful falls and injuries.

**Generalized atonic seizures** manifest with sudden loss or diminution of muscle tone ranging in severity from falls to only head nodding. Recovery is usually immediate, occurring within 1–2 s. In falls from the standing position, the patient suddenly flexes at the waist and knees, followed by further knee flexion, and then drops straight down and lands on the buttocks. When sitting, the patient falls forward or backward depending on the position of the centre of gravity. Consciousness is usually intact. However, longer atonic seizures with loss of consciousness do occur; the patient falls down and remains mute and motionless.

## What Is Status Epilepticus?

The duration of epileptic seizures is usually brief for seconds to 3–4 min and then they stop spontaneously. Status epilepticus is when epileptic seizures fail to terminate and last for more than 30 min. Any type of epileptic seizures can enter into status epilepticus. Generalized convulsive status epilepticus is the most severe of them that may cause cerebral damage and endanger life.

## Are There Any Precipitating and Facilitating Factors to Trigger Epileptic Seizures?

Epileptic seizures usually occur spontaneously without any precipitating factors. However, in some patients epileptic seizures are precipitated or facilitated by emotional factors, mental stress, excitement or frustration, fatigue or excessive alcohol or drug abuse [7]. Typical example of seizures precipitated by these factors is juvenile myoclonic epilepsy (see Chap. 8).

## Reflex Seizures

Some patients have reflex seizures. These are seizures which occur in direct response to certain stimuli such as:

Visual stimuli (Flickering light, Patterns), Thinking, Music, Eating, Praxis (planned action), Somatosensory, Proprioceptive, Reading, Hot water, Startle.
Television and video-games are the commoner causes of reflex epileptic seizures.

## Pathophysiology (Abnormal Physiology) of Epileptic Seizures

The pathophysiological mechanisms of epileptic seizures consist of evolving processes that are multiple, diverse and involve various levels of the functional organisation of the brain [8]. In simple terms seizures result from an imbalance between excitatory and inhibitory processes in the brain. Cellular excitability arises from mechanisms that affect cell membrane depolarization and repolarization. Abnormal synchronization of neuronal populations, propagation and termination of epileptic discharges involve more complex mechanisms most of which are currently unknown. Proposed mechanisms for the generation and spread of seizures include abnormalities in the ion channels, decreased inhibitory neurotransmission, or enhanced excitatory neurotransmission [8].

## Aetiology (Cause) of Epileptic Seizures

Any brain disorder that disturbs the structure or the function of the brain can cause epilepsy.

These include birth defects, brain tumours, infections, injuries, ischemia or anoxia, cerebrovascular disease, malformations of cortical development, chromosomal abnormalities, neurocutaneous disorders, degenerative brain disorders [5].

The inheritance of epilepsy is frequently complex. Some epilepsies such as Dravet syndrome are genetically determined; that means that certain genes can cause brain disorders that manifest with epileptic seizures alone or with other physical and mental symptoms. Specific genes have been identified in more than 20 different syndromes with epilepsy as a main feature. Many more single gene disorders that cause brain abnormalities or metabolic disorders manifest with epileptic seizures. Furthermore, the gene or genes that cause some epileptic syndromes have not yet been identified. Finally, some genetic disorders arise spontaneously through new gene mutations. Some people have a naturally low resistance to having seizures (a low 'seizure threshold') which can be in their genetic make-up.

## Epileptic Seizures That Are Not Considered as Epilepsy

In most definitions, epileptic seizures should be recurrent and unprovoked to constitute epilepsy. There are certain conditions with epileptic seizures that are traditionally not diagnosed as a form of epilepsy per se. These are:

A single epileptic seizure is not considered epilepsy unless further seizures occur.
Acute (provoked, occasional, reactive) symptomatic seizures are epileptic seizures
    that occur at the time with and as the result of an acute and transient brain disease
    or transient systemic disturbance. Such acute brain diseases are trauma, encepha-
    litis or cerebrovascular accident. Systematic disturbances include poisoning or
    drug overdose, alcohol or drug withdrawal, metabolic disorders or an electrolyte
    imbalance (such as uraemia, hyponatraemia, and hypoglycaemia).
Febrile seizures and benign neonatal seizures are also not considered as epilepsy

## Psychogenic Nonepileptic Seizures

Psychogenic seizures are non-epileptic events resembling an epileptic seizure, but without the characteristic electrical discharges associated with epilepsy. They looklike but they are not genuine epileptic seizures. They are stress-related or emotional and result from traumatic psychological experiences. They are sometimes called pseudoseizures or hysterical attacks but "psychogenic non-epileptic seizures" (PNES) is the accepted term [9].

Psychogenic nonepileptic seizures are common and frequently misdiagnosed as epilepsy. One in 5 of patients sent to epilepsy centres for difficult seizures is found to have Psychogenic nonepileptic seizures instead of epileptic seizures.

Their distinction from epileptic seizures is based on clinical history and manifestations and more definitely by recording them with video-EEG.

See Chap. 17 on psychogenic nonepileptic seizures.

## Recommendations for Patients with Epilepsy and Their Family

It is important to know what type of seizures you have because often the treatment differs from one to another type. It is also significant to recognize the symptoms of minor epileptic seizures because these define the affected area of the brain and may warn you on a forthcoming major convulsive seizure. For recommendations on the psychological and other aspects of epilepsy see Chaps. 17–25 of this book.

### What to Do When a Person Has a Generalized Tonic Clonic Seizure?

Generalized tonic clonic seizures usually end spontaneous after 2–3 min. What to do and what not to do during these convulsions is detailed in many epilepsy websites: Do place some clothing under the head to prevent injury; Do not try to restrain the person; Do not move the person unless they are in a dangerous place (for example next to a fire); do not place anything in the person's mouth (your fingers or a spoon); to prevent choking turn the head to the side.

Convulsive status epilepticus is when the convulsions do not terminate within a few minutes but continue for over 10 min to hours. This is a very serious and life threatening condition which requires urgent treatment in emergency hospital departments.

## Recommended Readings

- http://www.ilae.org/commission/class/diagnostic.cfm
  This is the ILAE Epilepsy Diagnosis.org which an excellent online diagnostic manual of the epilepsies, which provides information of how to diagnose seizure type(s), classify epilepsy, diagnose epilepsy syndromes and define the aetiology.
- https://www.epilepsy.org.uk/info/syndromes
  This is a detail guideline and support for patients with epilepsy in the Epilepsy Action which is the UK's leading epilepsy organisation.
- http://www.epilepsy.com/learn/types-epilepsy-syndromes
- http://www.epilepsy.com/information/professionals/about-epilepsy-seizures/overview-epilepsy-syndromes
  This is a detail guideline and support for patients with epilepsy in The Epilepsy Foundation of the USA and epilepsy,com.
- https://www.epilepsysociety.org.uk/what-epilepsy#.WE7PhPmLTIU
  This is a very useful website about epilepsy of the British Epilepsy Society.
- http://www.ncbi.nlm.nih.gov/books/NBK2606/
  This is the book "The epilepsies: Seizures, syndromes and management" provided by The National Center for Biotechnology Information.

## References

1. Fisher RS, van Emde BW, Blume W, Elger C, Genton P, Lee P, et al. Epileptic seizures and epilepsy: definitions proposed by the International League Against Epilepsy (ILAE) and the International Bureau for Epilepsy (IBE). Epilepsia. 2005;46:470–2.
2. Commission on Classification and Terminology of the International League Against Epilepsy. Proposal for revised clinical and electroencephalographic classification of epileptic seizures. Epilepsia. 1981;22:489–501.
3. Engel J Jr. Report of the ILAE classification core group. Epilepsia. 2006;47:1558–68.
4. Berg AT, Berkovic SF, Brodie MJ, Buchhalter J, Cross HJ, Van Emde Boas W, et al. Revised terminology and concepts for organization of seizures and epilepsies: Report of the ILAE Commission on Classification and Terminology, 2005-2009. Epilepsia. 2010;51:676–85.
5. Shorvon S, Perucca E, Engel J Jr, editors. The treatment of epilepsy. 3rd ed. Oxford: Willey-Blackwell; 2009.
6. Wyllie E, Cascino GD, Gidal B, Goodkin H, editors. The treatment of epilepsy. Principles and practice. 4th ed. Philadelphia: Lippincott Williams & Wilkins; 2006.

7.  Illingworth JL, Ring H. Conceptual distinctions between reflex and nonreflex precipitated sei-
    zures in the epilepsies: a systematic review of definitions employed in the research literature.
    Epilepsia. 2013;54:2036–47.
8.  Duncan JS, Sander JW, Sisodiya SM, Walker MC. Adult epilepsy. Lancet. 2006;367:1087–100.
9.  Valeta T. The potential of dramatherapy in the treatment of epilepsy. MA thesis, University of
    Derby; 2009.

# Febrile Seizures

**5**

**Abstract**

Febrile epileptic seizures are generalized convulsions precipitated by fever that is they are a specific response to any type of fever. They are common and often familial. They are either simple of good outcome or complicated with a 10% risk of developing epilepsy. A febrile convulsion is a dramatic experience to parents. Supportive family management and education are essential.

**Keywords**

Fever and epilepsy • Simple febrile convulsions • Complex febrile convulsions • Febrile convulsive status epilepticus • Treatment • Parental attitude • Parental education

## What Are Febrile Seizures? Clinical Manifestations

Febrile seizures or febrile convulsions are epileptic seizures precipitated by fever at 38 °C and above, they usually occur early in the course and may be the first apparent symptom of a febrile illness.

Generalized tonic-clonic convulsions are the commonest (90%) febrile seizures. In the more severe circumstances, the child suddenly loses consciousness, becomes unresponsive and stops breathing. Initially there is stiffening (contraction) of all body muscles (tonic convulsions) for a few seconds followed by violent and repetitive rhythmic clonic jerks (muscle tightening and relaxation) which last for 1–2 min. The child will fall, if standing, becomes blue, may pass urine, bite the tongue and vomit. Febrile seizures stop on their own, while the fever continues. When the convulsions stop, breathing starts again but the child is lethargic, drowsy and sleeps.

On rarer occasions, seizures consist of staring accompanied by stiffness or limpness, rhythmic jerking movements without prior stiffening, or focal stiffness or jerking only.

© Springer International Publishing AG 2017
T. Valeta, *The Epilepsy Book: A Companion for Patients*,
DOI 10.1007/978-3-319-61679-7_5

33

Febrile convulsions usually (92%) last for a few 3–6 min or less than 15 min. In the other one tenth, convulsions are longer than 15 min and two-thirds of these long seizures progress to febrile status epilepticus.

Sixteen percent of children is possible to have two or more febrile convulsions during the same febrile illness.

Because of different long-term risk (prognosis) significance, present practice subdivides febrile convulsions into:

- Simple febrile convulsions and
- Complex febrile seizures.

## Simple Febrile Convulsions

Simple febrile convulsions are generalized tonic-clonic lasting less than 15 min, and without recurrence within the next 24 h. They are the commoner type of 70% of all febrile convulsions.

## Complex Febrile Convulsions

Complex febrile convulsions (also known as "complicated" or "atypical") are defined by seizures that may be prolonged, repetitive or with focal features. One third of all febrile convulsions may have one, two or all three of these complicating factors.

- Prolonged are febrile convulsions of more than 15 min.
- Repetitive are febrile convulsions occurring in a cluster of 2 or more within 24 h.
- Focal febrile convulsions are those with focal (localized brain region) onset or those occurring in children with psychomotor (mental and motor) deficits caused in the perinatal period.

## What Is the Cause of Febrile Seizures? Aetiology-Genetics

Febrile convulsions are a specific response to any type of fever. Febrile seizures are often familial signifying genetic factors and predisposition. Febrile convulsions are at least two to three times more frequent in family members than in the general population.

## Febrile Illnesses Associated with Febrile Convulsions

The most commonly febrile illnesses are viral (90%) of upper respiratory tract infections, otitis media (infection of the middle ear), bronchopneumonia and gastrointestinal infection. Whooping cough, measles and meningitis were important causes when they were more common illnesses.

Seizures occurring soon after immunisation with diphtheria-pertussis-tetanus and measles vaccines are due to fever and not to the vaccine itself. Clinical presentation and generally benign outcome of these seizures is the same as of other febrile convulsions.

Children whose seizures are due to an infection of the brain and those who have had a previous afebrile seizure or central nervous system abnormality are not considered as febrile convulsions.

## What Makes a Child Prone (Predisposed) to Febrile Seizures? Risk Factors for a First or Recurrent Febrile Convulsions

The risk of a first febrile seizure is higher if there is a family history of other relatives with febrile seizures. The risk of younger siblings of affected children is around 10–20% and this is higher if a parent was also affected.

Males are more likely to be affected than females.

The risk of a recurrent febrile seizure is approximately two-fifths for any child with a first febrile seizure. Recurrence is most likely for those with

1. Early age at onset (less than 15 months).
2. Family history of febrile convulsions with a risk at 40–50%.
3. Short duration and low grade of temperature at the time of the first seizure.
4. Frequent numbers and high fever of subsequent febrile illnesses. Each new febrile episode increased the risk of recurrence by 18%.

## How Common Are Febrile Seizures and at What Age They Occur? Epidemiology

Febrile seizures occur in about ~3% of all children, Thus, approximately one in every 30 children will have at least one febrile seizure, and more than one-third of these children will have additional febrile seizures before they outgrow the tendency to have them.

Age of the child at first febrile seizure is between 6 months to 5 years with a peak at 18–22 months. The second half of the second year of life is the period that febrile convulsions are most likely to appear. Children rarely develop their first febrile seizure before the age of 6 months or after 3 years of age.

## How Febrile Seizures Are Diagnosed? Evaluation and Tests

A child with a febrile convulsion does not need any investigations other than detecting the cause of the fever. Febrile convulsions should be differentiated from 'seizures with fever' that include any seizure in any child with fever of any cause.

Accordingly, children with meningitis, encephalitis, or cerebral malaria do not have febrile seizures but have 'seizures with fever'.

A child who has a febrile seizure usually doesn't need to be hospitalized. If the seizure is prolonged or is accompanied by a serious infection, or if the source of the infection cannot be determined, a doctor may recommend that the child is admitted to the hospital for observation and management.

## Are Febrile Seizures Harmful? Psychomotor State

The vast majority of febrile seizures are not harmful. A febrile seizure does not seem to cause brain damage or affect the psychomotor status of the child. During a seizure, there is a small chance that the child may be injured by falling or may choke from food or saliva in the mouth. Using proper first aid for seizures can help avoid these hazards.

## What Is the Long Term Outcome (Prognosis) and Evolution?

Psychomotor development of children who were normal prior to the onset of febrile convulsions is normal. If psychomotor deficits, learning difficulties and behavioural problems are found in children with febrile convulsions, these are not related to febrile convulsions but probably reflect the overall developmental status of the child.

Overall, children with febrile convulsions have a six-fold excess (3%) of unprovoked seizures and subsequent epilepsy. The risk is 2% following a simple febrile seizure and 5–10% following a complex febrile seizure.

The risk is also increased for children with:

1. Abnormal neurological or development status such as cerebral palsy before first seizure
2. Family history of epilepsy

## What Is the Management of Febrile Seizures?

There is a 1999 USA practice parameter [1] and reviews [2–5] regarding the management of febrile convulsions.

## Acute Management of a Child with a Febrile Seizure

Control of the seizure is paramount. Treatment of the fever and mainly of the underlying illness is also important.

The majority of febrile seizures (80–90%) are brief and self-limited. They subside spontaneously within 2–5 min. The other 10–20% present with long-lasting convulsions, which are a genuine paediatric emergency that needs treatment as of convulsive status epilepticus.

## What a Parent Should Do for a Child Having a Febrile Seizure?

Early, usually parental, is more effective than late emergency treatment.

Seizures are frightening, but it is important that parents stay calm as much as possible and:

- To prevent accidental injury, the child should be placed on a protected safe surface such as the floor or ground, cannot fall down, injure or burn.
- To prevent choking, the child should be placed on his or her side or stomach and turn the head to the side.
- Watch for signs of breathing difficulty, including any color changes.
- Time the events. If the seizure lasts more than 5–10 min call for emergency assistance. This is especially urgent if the child shows symptoms of stiff neck, extreme lethargy, or abundant vomiting.
- If trained, administer a preparation of buccal (midazolam) or rectal (diastat) benzodiazepine for the termination of the seizure.
- When possible, gently remove any objects from the child's mouth.

Do not:

- Place anything in the child's mouth during a convulsion. Objects placed in the mouth can be broken and obstruct the child's airway.
- Do not try to hold or restrain the child.

For out of hospital administration of buccal midazolam or rectal diazepam, parents need specific training by the epilepsy nurse. See also instructions for

- Buccal midazolam in http://www.derbyshiremedicinesmanagement.nhs.uk/images/content/files/shared_care_guidelines/joint/Epistatus_Administer_DerbyPCT.pdf and
- Diastat in http://www.diastat.com/how-to-administer.aspx.

## Means of Lowering the Height of the Fever

Lowering temperature is to reduce discomfort of the febrile child and prevent dehydration.

Sponging with tepid water, antipyretics or both are usually recommended to reduce high fever.

## Prophylactic Management

### Simple Febrile Convulsions Do Not Need Prophylactic Treatment

The consensus for simple febrile seizures is that based on the risks and benefits of the effective therapies, neither continuous nor intermittent antiepileptic drug therapy is recommended for children with one or more simple febrile seizures. Recurrent episodes of febrile seizures can create anxiety in some parents and their children, and, as such, appropriate education and emotional support should be provided.

## Complex Febrile Convulsions May Occasionally Need Prophylactic Treatment

Prophylactic treatment may be desired if a child has one or mainly a combination of the following factors:

1. A focal or prolonged seizure,
2. Neurological abnormalities,
3. Age less than 1 year,
4. Multiple seizures occurring within 24 h
5. Frequent recurrences.

There are two options for prophylactic treatment in these cases:

- Continuous daily antiepileptic drug medication mainly with sodium valproate or phenobarbital.
- Intermittent treatment with diazepam or clobazam given only at the time of a febrile illness. Though opinions are divided of whether recurrences of febrile convulsions are prevented with this.

## Recommendations for Patients with Febrile Seizures and Their Family

Febrile convulsions, despite their excellent prognosis, are a dramatic experience of usually young age and inexperienced parents who often think that their child is dead or dying.

There is a need for supportive family management, education, and specific instructions about emergency procedures in possible subsequent seizures. Demonstrations of first aid practices for seizures are necessary, and parents must also be offered training to remain calm and confident about their child's seizures and condition.

Self-education is also important and this can be obtained through local epilepsy support groups, associations and reliable internet sources (see Chap. 26 on websites and other resources for people with epilepsy) [6].

Remember:

- Febrile seizures are always precipitated by fever 38 °C and above
- They are the most common type of seizure in children
- Onset is between 6 months to 5 years with a peak at 18–22 months
- One third of children have recurrences in subsequent febrile illnesses
- Prognosis is usually excellent. Psychomotor development is not affected.

- Febrile convulsions do not need EEG or MRI but the underlying cause of the fever should be thoroughly investigated.
- Though vigorous acute treatment of prolonged seizures is a medical emergency, prophylactic treatment is rarely needed.

## Recommended Readings

Febrile Seizures Fact Sheet in http://www.ninds.nih.gov/disorders/febrile_seizures/detail_febrile_seizures.htm
Febrile Seizures from NICE in http://cks.nice.org.uk/febrile-seizure#!topicsummary

## References

1. American Academy of Pediatrics. Practice parameter: long-term treatment of the child with simple febrile seizures. American Academy of Pediatrics. Committee on Quality Improvement, Subcommittee on Febrile Seizures. Pediatrics. 1999;103:1307–9.
2. Knudsen FU. Febrile seizures: treatment and prognosis. Epilepsia. 2000;41:2–9.
3. Dunlop S, Taitz J. Retrospective review of the management of simple febrile convulsions at a tertiary paediatric institution. J Paediatr Child Health. 2005;41:647–51.
4. Oluwabusi T, Sood SK. Update on the management of simple febrile seizures: emphasis on minimal intervention. Curr Opin Pediatr. 2012;24:259–65.
5. Offringa M, Newton R. Prophylactic drug management for febrile seizures in children (review). Evid Based Child Health. 2013;8:1376–485.
6. Valeta T. Parental needs of children with epileptic seizures and management issues. In: Panayiotopoulos CP, editor. Volume 1: a practical guide to childhood epilepsies. Oxford: Medicinae; 2006. p. 196–201.

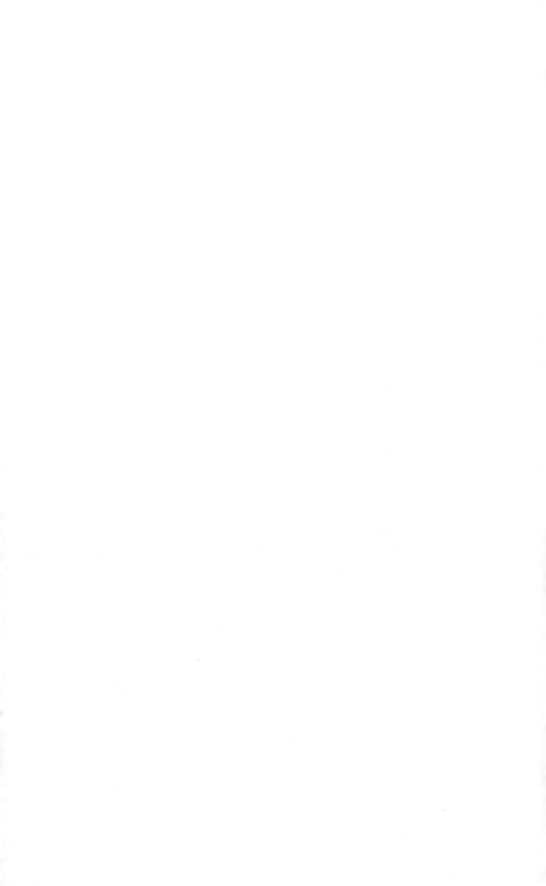

# Reflex Seizures

**6**

**Abstract**

Reflex seizures are those triggered by a specific stimulus which is characteristic for every one patient. Stimuli may come from the environment or from within the body. Photosensitive epilepsy is the commonest form of reflex epilepsy induced by flickering lights, television, video-games and discotheque lights. Some patients may have both reflex and spontaneous seizures. In epilepsy with reflex seizures only, avoiding the exposure to the triggering stimulus, often results to freedom of seizures without antiepileptic medication.

**Keywords**

Precipitated seizures • Triggered seizures • Television epilepsy • Video-game epilepsy • Self-induced seizures • Genetics

## What Are Reflex Seizures? Clinical Manifestations

Reflex epileptic seizures are those that are consistently caused by a specific stimulus which is characteristic for every one patient and may be environmental, internal or both [1–4]. The stimulus can be something simple in the environment such as flashes of light or more complex such as reading. Internal stimuli (from within the body) are also simple such as movement, or complex, such as thinking or decision-making.

Reflex seizures may be:

1. generalized, such as absences, myoclonic jerks, generalized tonic clonic seizures; or
2. focal, such as visual, motor or sensory seizures.

Some patients may have reflex seizures only but others may have both reflex and spontaneous seizures. Spontaneous seizures are those that occur out of the blue without apparent triggering (precipitating) factors.

## What Are the Triggers of Common Reflex Seizures?

Photosensitive epilepsy is the most common form of reflex epilepsy induced by flickering lights, television, video-games and discotheque lights as the main precipitating factors.

Seizures are more likely to occur from television when the patient is watching from close distance and particular programmes with flickering lights (usually a warning is issued in advance when the programme contains flickering lights).

Seizures are more likely to occur with video-games to patients who are sensitive to lights or patterns particularly after playing for long periods, when tired and sleep deprived.

Some types of reflex epilepsy are genetically determined.

Photosensitive epilepsy usually begins in childhood or early teenage. Often there is a family history of the same reflex seizures that is they are genetically determined. For the genetics of reflex epilepsy see at: https://www.orpha.net/data/patho/GB/uk-GeneticReflexEpilepsies.pdf

Patients are otherwise normal.

## What Are Self-Induced Seizures?

Some patients deliberately provoke seizures to themselves with techniques (manoeuvres) aiming to produce best conditions of stimulation by flickering light (self-induced photosensitive epilepsy), patterns (self-induced pattern-sensitive epilepsy), or higher brain functions (self-induced noogenic epilepsy). One manoeuvre for self-induction in photosensitive epilepsy is looking at a bright light source, usually the sun, and voluntarily waving the abducted fingers in front of the eyes (sunflower syndrome). Other techniques are: repetitive opening and closing of the eyes or lateral or vertical rhythmic movements of the head in front of a bright light source; making the television picture roll; quickly changing television channels while watching from a close distance; and playing video games.

The objective of self-induced seizures is relief of tension and anxiety, and escape from a disturbing situation.

## How Reflex Seizures Are Diagnosed?

Reflex seizures are diagnosed by history, recognizing the precipitating factors and confirmation with EEG.

## What Is the Long Term Outcome (Prognosis) and Evolution?

Prognosis is usually good but varies significantly in accordance with the underlying disease. It may be excellent with only one clinical epileptic seizure or be severe with continuing lifelong seizures. Photosensitivity generally declines after the age of 30–40 years.

## What Is the Treatment of Reflex Seizures?

The best management is with avoidance of precipitating factors. However, avoidance of precipitating factors may be impossible for patients with self-induced seizures who need psychiatric or psychological interventions.

AED treatment is usually needed for patients with reflex and spontaneous seizures.

## Recommendations for Patients with Epilepsy and Their Family

Not every seizure that happens in the presence of a particular stimulus is necessarily a reflex seizure because this could be a coincidence.

If you suspect that your seizures are triggered by a specific stimulus such as flickering lights, television or video-games take details of the events and your relation to the stimulus (distance for example) at the time that this happened and what you experienced.

A thorough family history is needed to find out whether other members have similar seizures, reflex or spontaneous.

In pure reflex epilepsy, avoiding the exposure to the triggering stimulus, often results to freedom of seizures without antiepileptic medication.

## Recommended Readings

- Reflex Seizures and Reflex Epilepsies at: https://www.ncbi.nlm.nih.gov/books/NBK2596/
- Reflex Epilepsy at http://emedicine.medscape.com/article/1187259-overview#showall
- Genetics of reflex epilepsies at: https://www.orpha.net/data/patho/GB/uk-GeneticReflexEpilepsies.pdf

## References

1. Panayiotopoulos CP. Reflex seizures and related epileptic syndromes. In: A clinical guide to epileptic syndromes and their treatment (Revised 2nd edition). London: Springer; 2010. p. 497–531.

2. Koepp MJ, Caciagli L, Pressler RM, Lehnertz K, Beniczky S. Reflex seizures, traits, and epilepsies: from physiology to pathology. Lancet Neurol. 2016;15:92–105.
3. Irmen F, Wehner T, Lemieux L. Do reflex seizures and spontaneous seizures form a continuum?—triggering factors and possible common mechanisms. Seizure. 2015;25:72–9.
4. Illingworth JL, Ring H. Conceptual distinctions between reflex and nonreflex precipitated seizures in the epilepsies: a systematic review of definitions employed in the research literature. Epilepsia. 2013;54:2036–47.

# Epileptic Syndromes and Their Classification

**7**

## Abstract

The recognition of epileptic syndromes is the most important milestone in modern epileptology because it allows accurate diagnosis and management of epilepsy. An epileptic syndrome, is a complex of clinical features, signs, and symptoms that together define a distinctive, recognizable clinical disorder. There are many types of epileptic syndromes which are grossly divided according to their type of epileptic seizures and their cause: A diagnosis of "epilepsy" or "seizures" should not be accepted without asking "what type/syndrome of epilepsy?" Then you make yourself aware of what this syndrome means and what it involves by appropriate questions to health careers and self-education.

### Keywords

Epilepsy syndrome • Diagnosis • ILAE • International League against Epilepsy • Electroclinical syndrome • Idiopathic • Symptomatic • Cryptogenic • Genetic • Structural • Metabolic • Immune • Infectious epilepsy

## What Is an Epileptic Syndrome?

There are many different types of epilepsy. The diagnosis of an epilepsy syndrome, includes factors such as the type of seizure the patient is having, severity and frequency of seizures, localization in the brain, age at seizure onset, cause, brain electrical features, physical or mental symptoms and signs, prognosis and response to treatment [1–5].

Formal definitions of epileptic syndromes by the International League against Epilepsy (ILAE) are:

Epileptic syndrome is an epileptic disorder characterized by a cluster of signs and symptoms, which customarily occur together; these include the type of seizure, aetiology, anatomy, precipitating factors, age of onset, severity, chronicity, diurnal and circadian cycling, and sometimes prognosis. However, in contradistinction to a disease, a syndrome does not necessarily have a common aetiology and prognosis. Epilepsy disease is a pathological condition with a single, specific, well defined aetiology [1].

The more recent formal ILAE definition is:

An electroclinical syndrome, is a complex of clinical features, signs, and symptoms that together define a distinctive, recognizable clinical disorder. These are distinctive disorders identifiable on the basis of a typical age onset, specific EEG characteristics, seizure types, and often other features which, when taken together, permit a specific diagnosis. The diagnosis in turn often has implications for treatment, management, and prognosis. These often become the focus of treatment trials as well as of genetic, neuropsychological, and neuroimaging investigations [2].

## What Is the Significance of Epileptic Syndrome Diagnosis?

The recognition of epileptic syndromes and diseases is the most important milestone in modern epileptology because it allows accurate diagnosis and management of seizure disorders.

Classifying epilepsy by seizure type alone leaves out other important information about the patient and the episodes themselves. A diagnosis limited to either epilepsy or seizures, is entirely unsatisfactory because this cannot provide guidance on important issues such as severity of the disease, prognosis, short- and long-term therapeutic decisions, and genetics (research and counselling), which are all factors that crucially affect personal, family and social life, education and career choices of patients. Defining the type of epilepsy should now be considered mandatory as it offers the best guide to both management and prognosis. Most epileptic syndromes and diseases are well defined and relatively easy to diagnose.

## What Types of Epileptic Syndromes Exist?

There are many types of epileptic syndromes (Table 7.1) which are grossly divided according to.

(a)  their type of epileptic seizures and
(b)  their aetiology (cause):

**Table 7.1** Electroclinical syndromes arranged by age at onset as proposed in the 2010 ILEA Organization for Epilepsy [2]

| |
|---|
| *Neonatal period* |
| Benign familial neonatal epilepsy (BFNE) |
| Early myoclonic encephalopathy (EME) |
| Ohtahara syndrome |
| *Infancy* |
| Epilepsy of infancy with migrating focal seizures |
| West syndrome |
| Myoclonic epilepsy in infancy |
| Benign infantile epilepsy |
| Benign familial infantile epilepsy |
| Dravet syndrome |
| Myoclonic encephalopathy in nonprogressive disorders |
| *Childhood* |
| Febrile seizures plus (can start in infancy) |
| Panayiotopoulos syndrome |
| Epilepsy with myoclonic atonic seizures |
| Benign epilepsy with centrotemporal spikes (Rolandic epilepsy) |
| Autosomal-dominant nocturnal frontal lobe epilepsy |
| Late onset childhood occipital epilepsy (Gastaut type) |
| Epilepsy with myoclonic absences |
| Lennox-Gastaut syndrome |
| Epileptic encephalopathy with continuous spike-and-wave during sleep |
| Landau-Kleffner syndrome |
| Childhood absence epilepsy |
| *Adolescence—Adulthood* |
| Juvenile absence epilepsy |
| Juvenile myoclonic epilepsy |
| Epilepsy with generalized tonic–clonic seizures alone |
| Progressive myoclonus epilepsies |
| Autosomal dominant epilepsy with auditory features |
| Other familial temporal lobe epilepsies |
| *Less specific age relationship* |
| Familial focal epilepsy with variable foci (childhood to adult) |
| Reflex epilepsies |
| *Others* |
| Mesial temporal lobe epilepsy with hippocampal sclerosis |
| Rasmussen syndrome |
| Gelastic seizures with hypothalamic hamartoma |
| Hemiconvulsion–hemiplegia–epilepsy |

## Epileptic Syndromes According to the Type of Epileptic Seizures

1. Generalized epileptic syndromes manifest themselves with any type of generalized epileptic seizures (absences, generalized tonic-clonic, tonic or clonic and myoclonic seizures).
2. Focal epileptic syndromes manifest with any type of focal epileptic seizures (motor, sensory, visual, cognitive etc).
3. Undetermined epileptic syndromes manifest with epileptic seizures of undetermined onset (focal or generalized).

## Epileptic Syndromes According to Aetiology

1. Idiopathic epilepsy syndrome is a syndrome that is only epilepsy, with no underlying structural brain lesion or other neurological signs or symptoms. These are presumed to be of genetic origin and are usually age dependent.
2. Symptomatic epilepsy syndrome is a syndrome in which the epileptic seizures are the result of one or more identifiable structural lesions of the brain.
3. Cryptogenic or probably symptomatic epilepsy syndrome is synonymous with, but preferred to, the term 'cryptogenic', used for defining syndromes that are believed to be symptomatic but no aetiology has been identified [1].

However, these terms of idiopathic, symptomatic and cryptogenic are no longer recommended by the 2010 ILAE Commission [2] which proposes the following concerning the aetiology of epilepsy in general:

(a) Genetic Epilepsies which are the direct result of a known or presumed genetic defect(s) in which seizures are the core symptom of the disorder. The genetic defect may arise at a chromosomal or molecular level. It is important to emphasize that "genetic" does not mean the same as "inherited" as de novo mutations are not uncommon. Having a genetic etiology does not preclude an environmental contribution to the epilepsy. (1) Chromosomal abnormalities such as in Angelman syndrome and (2) Gene abnormalities such as in Dravet syndrome
(b) Structural Epilepsies which are the result of distinct structural brain abnormality of any type
(c) Metabolic Epilepsies which are due to distinct metabolic abnormality.
(d) Immune Epilepsies which are due to a distinct immune-mediated aetiology with evidence of central nervous system inflammation. Rasmusen Syndrome is an example of immune epilepsy.
(e) Infectious Epilepsies which are of the commonest aetiology for epilepsy worldwide, especially in developing countries. Examples include tuberculosis, HIV, cerebral malaria, neurocysticercosis, cerebral toxoplasmosis.
(f) Unknown Aetiology Epilepsies which have an unkown underlying cause of the epilepsy.

Aetiology is also broken into six subgroups as above selected because of their potential therapeutic consequences in the new classification 2017 [6]. This classification incorporates aetiology along each stage (epileptic seizure, type of epilepsy, syndrome) emphasizing the need to consider aetiology at each step of diagnosis, as it often carries significant treatment implications. Aetiology is broken into six subgroups, selected because of their potential therapeutic consequences [6].

It is worth mentioning, that according to the 2006 ILAE proposal there are "special syndromes with seizures that are not diagnosed as a form of epilepsy" [1]:

1. febrile seizures
2. isolated seizures or isolated status epilepticus
3. benign neonatal seizures
4. seizures occurring only when there is an acute metabolic or toxic event due to factors such as alcohol, drugs, eclampsia [1].

Benign epilepsy syndrome (now called self-limited) is also a term commonly used for syndromes characterized by epileptic seizures that are age limited (neonates, infants and children) are easily treated or require no treatment and remit without sequelae. See Chap. 24.

## Recommendations to Patients with Epilepsy and Their Family

The significance of establishing a correct syndromic diagnosis should not be underestimated. This is because a number of important issues such cause, severity, outcome and treatment are often entirely different amongst syndromes of epilepsy (see for example rolandic epilepsy versus Rasmussen syndrome or juvenile myoclonic epilepsy). A diagnosis of "epilepsy" or "seizures" should not be accepted without asking "what type/syndrome of epilepsy?". It is fully legitimate and well understood a request for such syndromic diagnosis for you or your child from your caring physician. Then you make yourself aware of what this syndrome means and what it involves by appropriate questions to health carers and education through reading from the recommended appropriate interned sites (see below).

Also be aware that your doctor might be using the old definitions or the new ones which have been proposed in 2010 and again in 2017. New definitions have been introduced because a group of researchers in epilepsy felt that the classification or approach to this disease should change. This should not worry you. The epilepsies have not changed. There are different types of epilepsy and epilepsy syndromes and there may be different wording to describe them. You can ask your doctor and after you get an answer by him you can also look it up in this book for more information.

## Recommended Readings

- http://www.ilae.org/commission/class/diagnostic.cfm
  This is the ILAE EpilepsyDiagnosis.org which an excellent online diagnostic manual of the epilepsies.which provides information of how to diagnose seizure type(s), classify epilepsy, diagnose epilepsy syndromes and define the etiology.
- https://www.epilepsy.org.uk/info/syndromes
  This is a description of epileptic syndromes in the Epilepsy Action which is the UK's leading epilepsy organisation.
- http://www.epilepsy.com/learn/types-epilepsy-syndromes
- http://www.epilepsy.com/information/professionals/about-epilepsy-seizures/overview-epilepsy-syndromes
  This is a description of epileptic syndromes in The Epilepsy Foundation of the USA and epilepsy.com.
- http://www.ncbi.nlm.nih.gov/books/NBK2606/
  This is the book "The epilepsies: Seizures, syndromes and management" provided by The National Center for Biotechnology Information.

## References

1. Engel J Jr. Report of the ILAE classification core group. Epilepsia. 2006;47:1558–68.
2. Berg AT, Berkovic SF, Brodie MJ, Buchhalter J, Cross HJ, Van Emde Boas W, et al. Revised terminology and concepts for organization of seizures and epilepsies: Report of the ILAE Commission on Classification and Terminology, 2005-2009. Epilepsia. 2010;51:676–85.
3. Engel J Jr, Pedley TA, editors. Epilepsy: a comprehensive textbook. 2nd ed. Philladelphia: Lippincott William & Wilkins; 2008.
4. Wyllie E, Cascino GD, Gidal B, Goodkin H, editors. The treatment of epilepsy. Principles and practice. 4th ed. Philadelphia: Lippincott Williams & Wilkins; 2006.
5. Panayiotopoulos CP. A clinical guide to epileptic syndromes and their treatment (Revised 2nd edition). London: Springer; 2010.
6. Scheffer IE, Berkovic S, Capovilla G, Connolly MB, French J, Guilhoto L, et al. ILAE classification of the epilepsies: position paper of the ILAE Commission for Classification and Terminology. Epilepsia. 2017;58(4):512–21.

# Idiopathic Generalized Epilepsies

8

**Abstract**

Syndromes of idiopathic generalized epilepsy manifest with typical absences, myoclonic jerks and generalized tonic clonic seizures. A patient may have only one of these types of seizure but others may have a combination of two or all of them depending on syndrome. Patients are typically otherwise normal and have no anatomical brain abnormalities. Most syndromes of IGE start in childhood or adolescence, but some have an adult onset. The EEG is the most sensitive test in confirming the diagnosis. Response to appropriate antiepileptic drug is usually good but treatment may often be life-long.

**Keywords**

Childhood absence epilepsy • Juvenile absence epilepsy • Juvenile myoclonic epilepsy • EEG • Precipitating factors • Antiepileptic drugs

## What Are Idiopathic Generalized Epilepsies? Clinical Manifestations

Idiopathic generalized epilepsies (IGE) manifest with typical absences, myoclonic jerks and generalized tonic clonic seizures (see Chap 4 on epileptic seizures). A patient may have only one of these types of seizure but others may have a combination of two or all of them depending on syndrome. Absence status epilepticus is common. IGE are common and affect both sexes and all races. Patients are typically otherwise normal and have no anatomical brain abnormalities. Most syndromes of IGE start in childhood or adolescence, but some have an adult onset. They are usually lifelong though a few decline or stop with age. The EEG is the most sensitive test in confirming the diagnosis [1–3].

© Springer International Publishing AG 2017
T. Valeta, *The Epilepsy Book: A Companion for Patients*,
DOI 10.1007/978-3-319-61679-7_8

## What Are Syndromes of Idiopathic Generalized Epilepsy?

Syndromes of idiopathic generalized epilepsy are: [1]

- myoclonic epilepsy in infancy
- epilepsy with myoclonic-atonic seizures (also known as Doose syndrome)
- epilepsy with myoclonic absences
- childhood absence epilepsy
- juvenile absence epilepsy
- juvenile myoclonic epilepsy
- idiopathic epilepsy with generalized tonic clonic seizures alone.

I mainly describe in this chapter the most common of these syndromes such as childhood absence epilepsy, juvenile absence epilepsy and juvenile myoclonic epilepsy.

**Childhood absence epilepsy** (also known as petit mal epilepsy or pykno-lepsy) manifests exclusively with typical absence seizures in their most characteristic form. They are severe and frequent, tens or hundreds per day. They are of abrupt onset and abrupt termination, lasting from 4 to 20 s (mainly about 10 s). The hallmark of the absence is severe impairment of consciousness with unresponsiveness and interruption of the ongoing voluntary activity, often with a blank stare. If the patient is speaking, speech is slowed or interrupted; if walking, he or she stands transfixed. Usually the patient will be unresponsive when spoken to. Automatisms (involuntary movements such as lip licking, smacking, swallowing) occur in two-thirds of seizures, but are not stereotyped. Mild myoclonic elements of eyes, eyebrows and eyelids may feature at the onset of the absence. Absences are nearly invariably provoked by hyperventilation (deep and fast breathing) [1–3].

Other than absences, types of seizure are incompatible with childhood absence epilepsy (CAE) except febrile seizures and one or infrequent GTCS that may occur in adolescence after absences have stopped.

**Juvenile absence epilepsy** also manifests with severe typical absence seizures which are milder than those of childhood absence epilepsy. Generalized tonic clonic seizures are usually infrequent, and occur mainly after awakening from sleep particularly if the patient is sleep deprived. Myoclonic jerks if they occur, are mild and of random distribution.

**Juvenile myoclonic epilepsy** manifests with myoclonic jerks mainly on awakening, generalized tonic clonic seizures occurring usually after a series of myoclonic jerks and very mild (often undetectable) absences. Myoclonic jerks are shock-like, irregular, clonic-twitching movements. They affect eyelids, facial and neck muscles, upper more than lower limbs and body. They may be mild or violent that may make the patient fall on the ground, drop or throw things or kick. The patient is usually fully aware of myoclonic jerks. Precipitating (triggering) factors are sleep deprivation, fatigue, excitement or distress, alcohol excess and often flickering lights [1–3].

**Idiopathic epilepsy with GTCS alone** manifests only with generalized tonic clonic seizures. These mainly occur after awakening from sleep particularly if the patient is sleep deprived.

## What Is the Cause of Idiopathic Generalized Epilepsy? Aetiology/Genetics

Idiopathic generalized epilepsy is genetically determined (determined by the genes of an individual), as indicated by the high incidence of similar disorders amongst families. However, the precise mode of how these are inherited and the genes involved remain largely unknown.

## How Common Are Idiopathic Generalized Epilepsies and at What Age They Occur? Epidemiology

Idiopathic generalized epilepsies are very common. Thus, one third (30%) of patients with epilepsy have a type of IGE [1–3].

Childhood absence epilepsy affects around one out of ten children with epilepsy. It starts before the age of 10 (mainly around 5–6) years.

Juvenile myoclonic epilepsy occurs in 8–10% among patients with epilepsies. Commonly, it starts with myoclonic jerks in teenage (this is why it is called juvenile). GTCS start months after the onset of myoclonic jerks. However, absence seizures may in some children start earlier than myoclonic jerks and GTCS (7 years).

## How Are Idiopathic Generalized Epilepsies Diagnosed? Evaluation and Tests

IGE is usually diagnosed on good clinical description of the attacks (see Chaps. 3 and 14). The EEG is the most sensitive test for their diagnosis. This often reveals abnormalities which are typical when absences or myoclonic jerks occur. Absences are usually elicited when the child is asked to breath deep and fast.

Other tests such as brain scans are not needed but may be asked if the diagnosis is uncertain.

## What Is the Long Term Outcome (Prognosis) and Evolution

Childhood absence epilepsy usually declines and often stops after the age of 15 years when medication is gradually withdrawn.

All other types of IGE are probably lifelong, although patients show improvement after 40 years of age. It should be emphasized that severity of IGE varies amongst individuals. Some may have only a mild form with myoclonic jerks and rare GTCS particularly if they violate the precipitating factors. Other patients may have more severe forms with frequent and severe falls and GTCS. Seizures are generally well controlled with appropriate medication in up to 90% of patients.

## What Is the Management of Idiopathic Generalized Epilepsies?

Avoidance of seizure triggering factors and adherence to long-term medication is essential to prevent seizures. Advice with regard to the occurrence of seizures usually on awakening, lifestyle and seizure precipitants are very important. Sleep deprivation means staying very late at night and waking up after 4–5 h of sleep. Sleeping longer the next morning may well compensate staying up late at night. Photosensitive patients could prevent a seizure by covering one eye with the palm of the hand when in the presence of flickering lights (discothèques, television).

### Prophylactic Management

Most IGE respond well to appropriate antiepileptic drugs (valproate, levetiracetam, lamotrigine, ethosuximide, clonazepam); nearly all other antiepileptic drugs are contraindicated because they may aggravate seizures or be ineffective [4].

### How Long Should the Patient Continue Taking Antiepileptic Drugs?

With the exception of childhood absence epilepsy the syndromes of idiopathic generalized epilepsy need continuing medication even for many years after a seizure free period. The usual advice in epilepsy that withdrawal of medication should be attempted after 2–3 years from the last seizure is not good for idiopathic generalized epilepsy because relapses (reappearance of seizures) are common. However, if seizures were mild, infrequent and mainly occurring in the presence of precipitating factors drug withdrawal may be attempted. This should be in small decrements, probably over years. However, be aware that re-appearance of even minor seizures such as absences or myoclonic jerks mandates continuation of treatment. Video-EEG monitoring may be needed [1].

In childhood absence epilepsy treatment may be slowly withdrawn 2–3 years after controlling all absences.

### Recommendations for Patients with Epilepsy and Family

The anxiety and uncertainties of parents and patients with IGE is understandable [5]. This can be alleviated with proper education and knowledge on what is the particular syndrome, its prognosis and management. It is relieving to know that the majority of patients do well with little or any limitations in their life. The patient is usually fully aware of his/her myoclonic jerks. A significant part of your contribution is to understand the precipitating factors and help your children to deal with them [5].

Remember that:

- Idiopathic generalized epilepsies are common, one-third of all epilepsies
- They mainly start in childhood or adolescence
- They affect otherwise normal people of both sexes and all races
- They manifest with typical absences, myoclonic jerks and generalized tonic clonic seizures
- Seizures are usually spontaneous but they are also precipitated by sleep deprivation and some by environmental stimuli (flickering lights)
- The EEG is the most sensitive test in the confirmation of diagnosis

## Recommended Readings

- Epilepsy action at https://www.epilepsy.org.uk/info/syndromes/
- Epilepsy foundation at http://www.epilepsy.com/learn/types-epilepsy-syndromes/
- International League against Epilepsy at https://www.epilepsydiagnosis.org/syndrome/epilepsy-syndrome-groupoverview.html#
- Idiopathic Generalised Epilepsies at http://www.ncbi.nlm.nih.gov/books/NBK2608/

## References

1. Panayiotopoulos CP. The epilepsies: seizures, syndromes and management. Oxford: Bladon Medical Publishing; 2005.
2. Shorvon S, Perucca E, Engel J Jr, editors. The treatment of epilepsy. 3rd ed. Oxford: Willey-Blackwell; 2009.
3. Wyllie E, Cascino GD, Gidal B, Goodkin H, editors. The treatment of epilepsy. Principles and practice. 4th ed. Philadelphia: Lippincott Williams & Wilkins; 2006.
4. Beydoun A, D'Souza J. Treatment of idiopathic generalized epilepsy—a review of the evidence. Expert Opin Pharmacother. 2012;13:1283–98.
5. Valeta T. Parental needs of children with epileptic seizures and management issues. In: Panayiotopoulos CP, editor. A practical guide to childhood epilepsies, vol. 1. Oxford: Medicinae; 2006. p. 196–201.

# Benign Childhood Focal Epilepsy

**9**

## Abstract

Benign (or self-limited) childhood focal epilepsy affects otherwise normal children and includes three epileptic syndromes: rolandic epilepsy (or epilepsy with centrotemporal spikes), Panayiotopoulos syndrome and childhood occipital epilepsy of Gastaut. These syndromes affect 25% of children with non-febrile seizures. Epileptic seizures are focal with sensory-motor symptoms in rolandic epilepsy, autonomic symptoms in Panayiotopoulos syndrome, and visual/occipital lobe symptoms in childhood occipital epilepsy of Gastaut. EEG is very useful. Prophylactic treatment may not be needed. Parental education and psychological support is the most important aspect of management. All seizures stop usually in the mid-teens.

## Keywords

Rolandic epilepsy • Panayiotopoulos syndrome • Childhood occipital epilepsy of Gastaut • Centrotemporal spikes • Occipital spikes • Autonomic seizures

## What Is Benign Childhood Focal Epilepsy? Clinical Manifestations

Benign childhood focal epilepsy (self-limited or idiopathic focal epilepsy) affects otherwise normal children and includes three epileptic syndromes: [1, 2]

- rolandic epilepsy (or epilepsy with centrotemporal spikes) which is well known for over 70 years

© Springer International Publishing AG 2017
T. Valeta, *The Epilepsy Book: A Companion for Patients*,
DOI 10.1007/978-3-319-61679-7_9

- Panayiotopoulos syndrome, a common autonomic epilepsy, which is currently more readily diagnosed and
- idiopathic childhood occipital epilepsy of Gastaut, a less common form with uncertain prognosis.

In all patients seizures are focal (they start from one brain location).

## Rolandic Epilepsy

In rolandic epilepsy, seizures are focal and brief from 1 to 3 min. They manifest with:

- one sided (unilateral) facial sensory-motor symptoms which are often entirely localised in the lower lip or spread to the ipsilateral hand. Motor manifestations are sudden, continuous or bursts of jerks (clonic contractions), usually lasting from a few seconds to a minute. Sensory symptoms consist of unilateral numbness (tingling) mainly in the corner of the mouth.
- symptoms from inside the mouth, pharynx and larynx (oro-pharyngo-laryngeal symptoms) of strange sensations (tingling, prickling, freezing) and strange sounds, such as death rattle, gargling, grunting and guttural sounds.

These symptoms are often associated and occur together with hypersalivation (rivers of saliva in the mouth) and inability to speak (speech arrest) though the child is fully conscious.

In half of the children, these symptoms may progress to convulsions of one side of the body (hemiconvulsions) or both (generalized tonic clonic seizures).

Three-quarters of rolandic seizures occur during sleep.

## Panayiotopoulos Syndrome

In Panayiotopoulos syndrome, seizures are focal and often lengthy for over 6 min and almost half of them last for more than 30 min to many hours. Seizures commonly start with autonomic manifestations (see below), while consciousness and speech, as a rule, are preserved. Autonomic symptoms are mainly vomiting often together with skin pallor, incontinence, hypersalivation, breathing and heart rhythm irregularities. These are usually followed by deviation of the eyes, speech arrest, hemifacial convulsions and rarely visual hallucinations. Nearly always, the child gradually or suddenly becomes confused or unresponsive. One-third of seizures end with hemiconvulsions or generalized convulsions.

Nearly three-quarters of seizures occur during sleep.

## Idiopathic Childhood Occipital Epilepsy of Gastaut

In idiopathic childhood occipital epilepsy of Gastaut seizures primarily manifest with simple visual hallucinations, blindness or both. Visual hallucinations consist mainly of small multicoloured circular patterns. They are usually frequent, develop rapidly within seconds and are brief, lasting from a few seconds to 1–3 min. They may progress to convulsions. Headache is a frequent symptom after the end of the visual symptoms.

Seizures occur mainly while the child is awake and fully aware of them. Often these visual seizures are mistaken as migraine.

## What Is the Cause of Benign Childhood Focal Epilepsy? Aetiology-Genetics

Their cause is not known but genetic factors probably play a major role because there are often familial (occur in I the same family) within siblings and parents. The same child may have more than one type of benign childhood focal epilepsy. For example, seizures of Panayiotopoulos syndrome may appear first followed by rolandic seizures.

## How Common Are Benign Childhood Focal Seizures and at What Age They Occur? Epidemiology

They are the most common type of seizures in childhood. They affect 25% of children with non-febrile seizures.

Rolandic epilepsy is the commonest affecting around 15% of children aged 1–15 years with non-febrile seizures. In 75% of patients seizures start between 7 and 10 years.

Panayiotopoulos syndrome affects around 6% of children aged 1–15 years with non-febrile seizures. In 75% of patients seizures start between 3 and 6 years.

Idiopathic childhood occipital epilepsy of Gastaut is rarer accounting for about 2–7% of benign childhood focal seizures. Onset is between 3 and 15 years of age with a mean of around 8.

## How Are Benign Childhood Focal Seizures Diagnosed? Evaluation and Tests

The diagnosis is usually made on a good clinical history. Electroencephalography (EEG) is the most useful test. However, it may be re-assuring to also obtain a brain scan though this may not be needed in straightforward cases.

The abnormalities in the EEG are often characteristic and consist of frequent and severe spikes which are localized (focal) in the centrotemporal regions (rolandic epilepsy), occipital regions (occipital epilepsy) or many brain regions (Panayiotopoulos syndrome). These abnormalities increase during sleep. A first routine EEG may be normal in around 10% of the patients.

Severity of EEG does not predict outcome or severity of the disease.

## Are Benign Childhood Focal Seizures Harmful?

The vast majority of benign childhood focal seizures are not harmful. They do not seem to cause brain damage or affect the psychomotor status of the child. Even if seizures are prolonged as in Panayiotopoulos syndrome, neurological findings are unlikely to change.

During a seizure, there is a small chance that the child may be injured by falling or may choke from food, saliva or vomiting. Using proper first aid for seizures can help avoid these hazards. However, a small minority of children with Panayiotopoulos syndrome may develop during the seizure severe cardio-respiratory problems which may be life threatening.

## What Is the Long Term Outcome (Prognosis) and Evolution?

The prognosis for rolandic epilepsy and Panayiotopoulos syndrome is invariably excellent, with probably less than 2% risk of developing epilepsy in adult life. No more seizures (remission) occur within 2–4 years from onset and certainly before the age of 16 years. The total number of seizures is low, the majority of patients having fewer than ten seizures; 10–20% have just a single seizure. About 10–20% may have frequent seizures, but these also remit with age.

Children with rolandic epilepsy may develop usually mild and reversible linguistic, cognitive and behavioural abnormalities during the active phase of the disease. This is less likely to happen with Panayiotopoulos syndrome.

The development, social adaptation and occupations of adults with a previous history of benign childhood focal seizures is normal.

## What Is the Management of Benign Childhood Focal Seizures?

Parental education and psychological support is the most important aspect of management (see Chap. 24 on Psychosocial aspects—parental reactions and needs in idiopathic focal epilepsies) [3–5].

### Acute Management of Benign Childhood Focal Seizures

Control of the seizure is paramount. Long-lasting seizures (>10 min) or status epilepticus (>30 min–hours) (particularly common in Panayiotopoulos syndrome) is a genuine paediatric emergency that demands appropriate and vigorous diagnosis and treatment. Early, usually parental administration of appropriate drugs and mainly buccal midazolam is more effective than late emergency treatment. Aggressive treatment (particularly when intravenous lorazepam or diazepam are used) should be avoided because of the risk of complications, including cardiorespiratory arrest.

## What a Parent Should Do for a Child Having a Seizure?

Seizures are frightening, but it is important that parents stay calm as much as possible and:

- If the child is conscious, reassure him/her that everything should be fine
- Gently, move the child to a safe place to avoid injury or burn in case of convulsions
- To prevent choking, the child should be placed on his or her side or stomach and turn the head to the side.
- Watch for signs of breathing difficulty, including any color changes.
- Time the events. If the seizure lasts more than 5–10 min call for emergency assistance. This is especially urgent if the child shows symptoms of stiff neck, extreme lethargy, or abundant vomiting.
- If trained, administer a preparation of buccal (midazolam) or rectal (diastat) benzodiazepine for the termination of the seizure according to a prepared protocol by the physician
- When possible, gently remove any objects from the child's mouth.

Do not:

- place anything in the child's mouth during a convulsion. Objects placed in the mouth can be broken and obstruct the child's airway.
- Do not try to hold or restrain the child.

## Prophylactic Management

Prophylactic treatment with anti-epileptic medication is not recommended for rolandic epilepsy and Panayiotopoulos syndrome even for patients with lengthy seizures or more than two recurrences [6]. Although this may prevent the occurrence of additional seizures, potential adverse effects may not commensurate with the benefit. There is no increased risk of subsequent epilepsy or neurological deficit. Prophylactic treatment may be desired in idiopathic childhood occipital epilepsy, if a child has multiple recurrences or in the unlikely event of parental insistence. Though there is no evidence of superiority amongst monotherapy with various drugs most authors prefer carbamazepine or valproate.

There is no need to continue medication 1–3 years after the last seizure and certainly not after age 14 when most benign childhood focal seizures remit [6].

## Recommendations for Patients with Benign Childhood Focal Epilepsy and Their Family

I have documented that despite their excellent prognosis, benign childhood focal seizures usually have a dramatic impact to parents. In Chap. 24 Psychosocial aspects— parental reactions and needs you will find details of my research and results based on a questionnaire especially designed for parents of children with idiopathic focal epilepsy [3–5]. In my studies, the most dominant points of parental anxiety and concerns refer to their uncertainty of the nature, the cause and the impact of the events on their child's development as well as the lack of appropriate information. There is a need for supportive family management, education and specific instructions about emergency procedures for possible subsequent seizures. Education and psychological support is the cornerstone of the optimal management. Parents should be given general information about benign childhood focal seizures and Panayiotopoulos syndrome, in which seizures may have dramatic features and last for many hours; the situation is frequently compounded by physicians' uncertainty over diagnosis, management and prognosis. Parents who have watched their child during a seizure may need specific psychological support to overcome anxiety and panic that may result in overprotection and interfere in turn with parent–child separation and independence [3–5].

## Recommended Readings

- Benign Childhood Focal Seizures and Related Epileptic Syndromes at. http://www.ncbi.nlm.nih.gov/books/NBK2598/
- Epilepsy action at https://www.epilepsy.org.uk/info/syndromes/
- Epilepsy foundation at http://www.epilepsy.com/learn/types-epilepsy-syndromes/
- International League against Epilepsy at https://www.epilepsydiagnosis.org/syndrome/epilepsy-syndrome-groupoverview.html#

## References

1. Panayiotopoulos CP, Michael M, Sanders S, Valeta T, Koutroumanidis M. Benign childhood focal epilepsies: assessment of established and newly recognized syndromes. Brain. 2008;131:2264–86.
2. Panayiotopoulos CP, Bureau M, Caraballo RH, Dalla Bernardina B, Valeta T. Idiopathic focal epilepsies in childhood. In: Bureau M, Genton P, Dravet C, Delgado-Escueta AV, Tassinari CA, Thomas P et al., editors. Epileptic syndromes in infancy, childhood and adolescence, 5th ed. with video. Montrouge: John Libbey Eurotext; 2012; p. 217–254.
3. Valeta T. Psychosocial aspects, parental reactions and needs in idiopathic focal epilepsies. Epileptic Disord. 2016;18:19–22.
4. Valeta T. Parental reactions in benign childhood focal seizures. Epilepsia. 2012;53(Supplem 5):222–3.
5. Valeta T. Parental attitude, reaction and education in benign childhood focal seizures. In: Panayiotopoulos CP, editor. The epilepsies: seizures, syndromes and management. Oxford: Bladon Medical Publishing; 2005. p. 258–61.
6. Valeta T, Panayiotopoulos CP. Treatment of classic syndromes in idiopathic focal epilepsies in childhood. J Pediatr Epilepsy. 2016;5:142–6.

# Epileptic Encephalopathies

# 10

**Abstract**

Epileptic encephalopathies are severe diseases of the brain starting at an early age of childhood and more usually in infancy. They manifest with (1) frequent and various types of epileptic seizures which are resistant to treatment and (2) cognitive, behavioural and neurological deficits which often worsen with time (progressive). West, Lennox-Gastaut and Dravet syndrome are described in this chapter. In addition to addressing seizures, holistic care for patients with epileptic encephalopathies must involve a multidisciplinary team that includes specialists in psychotherapy, physical, occupational and speech therapy and social work. Families need significant and continuous multiple support.

**Keywords**

West syndrome • Lennox-Gastaut syndrome • Dravet syndrome • Cognitive decline • Psychological support • Treatment • SUDEP

## What Are Epileptic Encephalopathies? Clinical Manifestations

Epileptic encephalopathies are severe diseases of the brain starting at an early age of childhood and more usually in infancy. They manifest with: (1) frequent and various types of epileptic seizures which are resistant to treatment and (2) cognitive, behavioural and neurological deficits which often worsen with time (progressive) [1, 2].

Syndromes of epileptic encephalopathies are:

- early myoclonic encephalopathy
- Ohtahara syndrome
- West syndrome
- Dravet syndrome ('severe myoclonic epilepsy in infancy')
- Lennox-Gastaut syndrome

- epileptic encephalopathy with continuous spike-and-wave during sleep (in the EEG) including Landau–Kleffner syndrome
- myoclonic encephalopathy in non-progressive disorders

In this Chap. I detail West and Lennox-Gastaut syndrome which are more common. I also describe Dravet syndrome because of recent interest due to its genetic links, severity and increased mortality.

**West syndrome (infantile spasms)** is characterized with epileptic seizures called epileptic spasms. These are clusters of sudden, brief for a second or two, bilateral spasms (tonic contractions) of the body and limbs. They may involve the neck only (bobbing of the head), abdomen (mild bending) or just the shoulders (a shruglike movement). A cry may follow the end of the attack. The epileptic spasms happen on arousal from sleep and during alert states, less often during sleep. When the disease starts the epileptic spasms are usually mild and infrequent but in a few weeks they significantly worsen with 1–30 clusters per day and each cluster having 20–150 attacks.

**Lennox-Gastaut syndrome** is a severe form of epilepsy. Seizures usually begin before 4 years of age. Seizure types, which vary among patients, include tonic (stiffening of the body often with altered respiratory patterns), atonic (brief loss of muscle tone and consciousness, causing abrupt falls), atypical absence (staring spells), and myoclonic (sudden muscle jerks). The duration of seizures vary from brief (seconds to minutes) to very prolonged or non-stop status epilepticus. Seizures are common when the child is inactive and in sleep. There may be periods of prolonged and frequent, multiple times per day, seizures, mixed with brief, relatively seizure-free periods.

**Dravet syndrome** is a rare but very severe genetic epilepsy syndrome. The typical form develops in three stages. The first stage starts in the first year of life, with the occurrence of febrile and afebrile, generalized or unilateral, clonic seizures in apparently normal infants. The second stage follows later with the appearance of other seizure types of mainly massive myoclonus (myoclonic and atypical absence seizures, focal seizures, status epilepticus). The seizures are usually accompanied by a slowing of psychomotor development, cognitive impairment and behavioural disturbances. The third stage starts at around the age of 10 years with improvement in seizures but deteriorating gait, intellectual and other neurologic disabilities. The long-term prognosis is unfavourable and early death can occur due to SUDEP or to status epilepticus. Simply prescribing medication is inadequate to help families which need continuous support [3, 4].

## What Is the Cause of Epileptic Encephalopathies? Aetiology-Genetics

Most children with West syndrome have abnormal neurological and mental states which pre-exist the appearance of spasms and they are caused by a variety of brain lesions from or around the birth. Tuberous sclerosis is common.

Similarly, Lennox-Gastaut syndrome can be caused by numerous brain diseases but in one third of cases, no cause can be found [5].

Dravet syndrome is genetically determined. A mutation in the SCN1A gene is found in 70–80% of the patients [6].

## What Makes a Child Prone (Susceptible) to an Epileptic Encephalopathy?

This not known but it is assumed that the electrical (EEG) discharges and epileptic seizures are a specific reaction of the immature developing brain to any abnormality. This reaction manifests differently in neonates, infants and young children. It is also assumed that the psychomotor deficits and regression of the child are caused by the interruption of the normal maturation of the brain by the epileptic electrical and seizure activity.

## How Common Are Epileptic Encephalopathies and at What Age They Occur? Epidemiology

All epileptic encephalopathies mainly occur in early life.

Early myoclonic encephalopathy and Ohtahara syndrome occur in neonates.

West syndrome happens in 1 of every 4000 children. It is the most common type of epileptic encephalopathy. It usually starts at the age of 3–7 months; rarely before 3 months or after 1–5 years.

Lennox-Gastaut syndrome has a prevalence of 5–10% of children with epilepsy and starts between 1 and 7 years (peak 3 and 5 years). Half of the cases of West syndrome later develop Lennox-Gastaut syndrome.

Dravet syndrome is a rare disease with an incidence of less than 1 per 40,000. It starts in the first year of life.

## How Are Epileptic Encephalopathies Diagnosed? Evaluation and Tests

The confirmation of epileptic encephalopathies is with EEG. In West syndrome EEG shows severe abnormalities known as hypsarrhythmia. Commonly, typical are also the EEG abnormalities in Lennox-Gastaut syndrome (slow spike and wave and fast spikes).

However, a number of other tests (brain scans, blood, urine and, sometimes, spinal fluid tests) may be asked to identify the main cause. Molecular genetic testing is required for Dravet syndrome.

## Are Epileptic Encephalopathies Harmful?

Uncontrolled and frequent seizures and mainly status epilepticus are harmful to the brain and development of the child. They may also endanger life. Falls from seizures pose a serious risk of injury.

## What Is the Long Term Outcome (Prognosis) and Evolution?

Most of the children go on to develop significant epilepsy often with severe motor and mental disability. Only one out of ten patients has near normal development. Dravet syndrome has the worst prognosis.

However, all epileptic encephalopathies have a tendency to decline, discontinue or even stop in adolescence, but often with serious neurocognitive residual effects.

Behavioral problems are common, ranging from hyperactivity to autistic behaviors.

The outcome is likely to be best for children with an unknown cause compared to those whose seizures are caused by brain lesions (structural epilepsy).

## What Is the Management of Epileptic Encephalopathies?

Seizures in epileptic encephalopathies are usually intractable. Antiepileptic drugs may reduce them but do not control them, and it is doubtful if they affect the outcome [7–9]. Avoiding drugs that may cause drowsiness or worsen seizures, cognition, and behaviour is important.

Management is demanding and should include the following elements:

- Treatment of epileptic seizures with appropriate medications and nonpharmacological methods.
- Treatment of behavioural and cognitive problems with appropriate educational programs.
- Physical therapy for the patient's physical disabilities.
- Family support.

## Prophylactic Medication

In West syndrome, the antiepileptic drug vigabatrin or adrenocorticotropic hormone (ACTH) control the spasms in two-thirds of patients within days. Final outcome may not be influenced by treatment.

In Lennox-Gastaut syndrome, many anti-epileptic drugs are used. There is usually no single AED that will control seizures. Children who improve initially may later show tolerance (not respond) to a drug or have uncontrollable seizures. Ketogenic diet is highly beneficial in some cases. Neurosurgical interventions are now possible and effective in selected cases.

Dravet syndrome is among the most challenging diseases. Prophylactic medical management of seizures is usually inadequate. Ketogenic diet may be useful. Several agents in development may show promise [10]. Families must be counselled on non-pharmacologic strategies to reduce seizure risk.

Mozart's music is recommended for children with drug-refractory epileptic encephalopathies [11].

## Acute Management of Epileptic Encephalopathies

This falls into the general management of prolonged seizures and status epilepticus which is a medical emergency. These should be stopped as soon as possible. Early parental intervention with buccal midazolam or rectal diazepam is crucial (see status epilepticus).

## Recommendations for Parents of Children with Epileptic Encephalopathies

Parents of a child with an epileptic encephalopathy have difficult decisions and adaptations to make from the time of diagnosis and to the future. This refers to medical treatments, physical and cognitive management, educational, social and financial needs. It may be a lifelong challenge affecting many areas of life. The seizures are often difficult to control that can lead to frequent hospital admissions. Though epileptic encephalopathies do not have a cure, there are many ways to help the child in achieving the maximal of its potentials. Be prepared of what to do when an emergency occurs and seek ways of preventing them. Deep knowledge of the situation, what to expect and where to find the best medico-psycho-social assistance are of paramount importance.

- Get as much information from your health care professionals and educate yourself about the disease through books and the internet
- Register in a formal epileptic encephalopathy relevant website, join support groups and share questions and answers in e-communities with other people who are going through something similar. This can help alleviate some of the fear of unfamiliarity, gain valuable tips and advice and help your planning.
- Ask for a thorough assessment of your child's medical, cognitive and physical condition and planning for frequent follow up and emergencies.
- Investigate the availability of health care (state, insurance) for the child's health including emergency facilities.
- Obtain personal training in case of emergency (administration of drugs needed to terminate status epilepticus)
- For optimal care, some of these children require 24/7 monitoring by a caregiver. Find out whether you are eligible for such assistance either through the national health service or your insurance. Your child may also be eligible for an individualized education plan and services through the state school and health systems. Be aware that sometimes you have to fight hard against administrative difficulties and rigidity. There is an unmet need and gap in coordination of the care of these children
- Staff at the child's school, need to be aware of the child's condition and what to do in the event of an emergency. The school's Special Educational Needs Co-ordinator will usually be the person to go to about ensuring necessary arrangements and allowances are in place.

Remember:

- Epileptic encephalopathies are relatively rare but serious disorders in neonates, infants and younger children
- They manifest with frequent and various type of seizures and status epilepticus that are difficult to control as well as cognitive, behavioural and neurological deficits which often worsen with time (progressive)
- Most of these children have pre-existing brain abnormalities
- Most of the children go on to develop significant epilepsy often with severe motor and mental disability. Only one out of ten has near normal development.
- All epileptic encephalopathies have a tendency to decline, discontinue or even stop in adolescence, but often with serious neurocognitive residual effects.
- Management is demanding and often frustrating.

## Recommended Readings

- West syndrome foundation http://www.infantilespasmsinfo.org/index.php
- Lennox-Gastaut syndrome http://lgsfoundation.org/index.html
- Dravet syndrome http://www.dravetfoundation.org/dravet-syndrome/what-is-dravet-syndrome
- Intractable childhood epilepsy http://www.ice-epilepsy.org/vision-2020-task-force.html
- Epilepsy action at https://www.epilepsy.org.uk/info/syndromes/
- Epilepsy foundation at http://www.epilepsy.com/learn/types-epilepsy-syndromes/
- International League against Epilepsy at https://www.epilepsydiagnosis.org/syndrome/epilepsy-syndrome-groupoverview.html#
- Epileptic Encephalopathies in Infancy and Early Childhood at http://www.ncbi.nlm.nih.gov/books/NBK2611/

## References

1. Guerrini R, Pellock JM. Age-related epileptic encephalopathies. Handb Clin Neurol. 2012;107:179–93.
2. Covanis A. Epileptic encephalopathies (including severe epilepsy syndromes). Epilepsia. 2012;53(Suppl 4):114–26.
3. Wirrell EC, Laux L, Donner E, Jette N, Knupp K, Meskis MA, et al. Optimizing the diagnosis and management of Dravet syndrome: recommendations from a North American Consensus Panel. Pediatr Neurol. 2017;68:18–34.
4. Camfield P, Camfield C, Nolan K. Helping families cope with the severe stress of Dravet syndrome. Can J Neurol Sci. 2016;43(Suppl 3):S9–S12.
5. McTague A, Howell KB, Cross JH, Kurian MA, Scheffer IE. The genetic landscape of the epileptic encephalopathies of infancy and childhood. Lancet Neurol. 2015;15:304–16.
6. Cetica V, Chiari S, Mei D, Parrini E, Grisotto L, Marini C, et al. Clinical and genetic factors predicting Dravet syndrome in infants with SCN1A mutations. Neurology. 2017;88:1037–44.

7. Vigevano F, Arzimanoglou A, Plouin P, Specchio N. Therapeutic approach to epileptic enceph-alopathies. Epilepsia. 2013;54(Suppl 8):45–50.
8. Covanis A. Clinical management of epileptic encephalopathies of childhood and infancy. Expert Rev Neurother. 2014;14:687–701.
9. Jehi L, Wyllie E, Devinsky O. Epileptic encephalopathies: optimizing seizure control and developmental outcome. Epilepsia. 2015;56:1486–9.
10. Wirrell EC. Treatment of Dravet syndrome. Can J Neurol Sci. 2016;43(Suppl 3):S13–8.
11. Coppola G, Toro A, Operto FF, Ferrarioli G, Pisano S, Viggiano A, et al. Mozart's music in children with drug-refractory epileptic encephalopathies. Epilepsy Behav. 2015;50:18–22.

# Structural (Symptomatic) Focal Epilepsy

**11**

**Abstract**

Structural (or symptomatic) epilepsy is any type of epilepsy caused by damage of brain structure for example injury, infection, tumours, anoxia, hereditary or metabolic diseases. Lesions may be the remaining of an old problem (residual) while others may get worse in time (progressive). The symptoms of epileptic seizures depend on the brain site of the lesion (frontal, parietal, temporal, occipital). Mesial temporal lobe epilepsy is the commoner type of structural epilepsy. The outcome depends on the underlying cause and the extent of the lesion. The needs of patients with structural epilepsy vary significant depending on the severity of epilepsy and the severity of brain damage.

**Keywords**

Frontal • Parietal • Temporal • Occipital epilepsy • Epigastric aura • Visual hallucinations • Deja vu • Automatisms • Brain MRI • Psychosocial needs Neurosurgical treatment

## What Is Structural Epilepsy? Clinical Manifestations

This is any type of epilepsy caused by structural or metabolic lesions of the brain. Ictal symptoms, particularly at onset, are determined by the localization (site) of the lesion in the brain irrespective of its cause (etiology). However, outcome and prognosis is mainly determined on the basis of aetiology rather than simply the site of the lesion in the brain (localization). Mesial temporal lobe epilepsy with hippocampal sclerosis is a striking example of this.

**Temporal lobe epilepsy** is the commoner type. Symptoms depend on whether the lesions are in the mesial (mainly hippocampal) or the lateral temporal lobe. Epigastric aura and fear are the commonest and often the initial manifestations of mesial temporal lobe seizures. Auditory hallucinations mainly characterize the lateral temporal lobe seizures. Déjà vu or jamais vu are common in both.

Epigastric aura is a strange sensation (like pain, emptiness, squeezing) felt around the bellybutton which within seconds moves upwards and when it reaches the neck the patient loses consciousness.

Déjà vu (already seen) is a feeling of overwhelming sense of familiarity with something that shouldn't be familiar at all.

Déjà vu and other symptoms are experienced by most normal people, their epileptic nature is suspected by the presence and the sequence of other epileptic events that may precede, coincide or follow them.

Automatisms (lip smacking, hand rubbing, walking around) are common manifestations of temporal lobe epilepsy. They are described by witnesses because the patient is unaware of them.

Postictal (after the end of the seizure) symptoms are common and include mental and physical fatigue, drowsiness, headache,  inability to concentrate and confusion.

**Frontal lobe epilepsy** has various manifestations depending on the localization of the lesion. When this is in the lateral aspect of the frontal lobe (motor area) there are clonic spasms of one thumb and one side of the face which may spread to the whole arm and one side of the body. When this is in the medial aspect of the frontal lobe, seizures mainly occur during sleep and consist of sudden bizarre bilateral, asymmetric body posturing and movements with frequent weird voices and sounds. These seizures are brief for seconds to a minute and may happen many times per night.

**Occipital lobe epilepsy** usually manifests with brief seizures of visual hallucinations which are often multicolored circles or balloons. They come suddenly within seconds and last for 1–2 min. Headache usually follows the end of the seizure. Occipital lobe seizures may be misdiagnosed for migraine though the visual aura of migraine starts slowly in minutes, last longer 15 min and presents with zigzag lines.

**Parietal lobe epilepsy** is often difficult to detect because seizures are predominantly sensory (tingling and a feeling of electricity, pain). They mainly affect one hand and one side of the face. Vertigo (mainly rotation) or disorientation in space may occur.

## What Is the Cause of Structural Epilepsy? Aetiology

Structural epilepsy can be caused by any type of lesion in the brain. Lesions may be due to anoxia (lack of oxygen to the brain) around birth, head injury of any reason, infections, cysts, abnormalities of brain development, hereditary diseases, degenerative disorders (progressive and deteriorating conditions, often associated with loss of brain cells), tumors, stroke and poisoning. There are significant variations between developed and developing countries. For example, cysticercosis and tuberculomas are among the commonest causes of epilepsy in developing countries, but have a minimal prevalence in Western industrialized countries.

Lesions may be the remaining of an old problem (residual) while others may get worse in time (progressive). For example residual is the damage caused in a road traffic accident while the damage caused by a brain tumor is progressive.

## What Makes a Patient with a Structural Brain Abnormality Prone to Epileptic Seizures?

Structural abnormalities of the brain disturb the normal communication and balances between nerve cells and this may cause epileptic seizures. However, only a relatively small number of patients with structural brain lesions develop epilepsy. This is because the level of sensitivity to develop epilepsy (threshold) varies significant amongst subjects depending on many factors and family history.

## How Common Is Structural Epilepsy and at What Age They Occur? Epidemiology

It is the commoner type of epilepsy. Probably two-thirds of epilepsy is caused by structural lesions of the brain. It starts at any age and affects both sexes. Mesial temporal lobe epilepsy accounts for around 20% of patients with epilepsy. Most of these patients had a history of prolonged febrile seizures.

## How Is Structural Epilepsy Diagnosed? Evaluation and Tests

Brain MRI is the main test to detect abnormalities of the brain. The EEG plays a less important role and may be normal. The treating physician may also request other specific appropriate blood or urine tests.

## Is Structural Epilepsy Harmful?

Some causes of structural epilepsy are harmful themselves because of their progressive nature (tumors for example). Epileptic seizures of structural epilepsy have the same risks as in any other type of epilepsy.

## What Is the Long Term Outcome (Prognosis) and Evolution?

This depends on the underlying cause and the extent of the lesion. Some may be mild without serious effects on the patient but others may be severe affecting physical and mental development. Similarly epileptic seizures may be infrequent and mild while others are frequent and severe. Around half of children with structural focal epilepsy become seizure free for many years [1].

## What Is the Management of Structural Epilepsy?

Treatment is of the underlying cause and of the epileptic seizures. The treatment of focal seizures begins first with appropriate antiepileptic drugs. With one drug around 30% of patients may become seizure free [2]. This is increased to 60% if treatment is with combined antiepileptic drugs [1]. If prophylactic treatment with AEDs fails, neurosurgical options are now becoming more widely available and are often life saving for some patients and particularly those with mesial temporal lobe epilepsy.

## How Long Should the Patient Continue Taking Antiepileptic Drugs?

It is possible that treatment is lifelong because of relapses when drugs are stopped. Many authorities recommend attempts of very slow withdrawal from AED in months [3] for patients who are free of seizures for at least 3–4 years. However, seizure-recurrence may have devastating, medical, psychological and social consequences for the individual, for example injury and loss of self-esteem. Also, it is reported that one in five patients does not re-enter remission and for some patients, it may take several years to become seizure-free again [3].

## Recommendations for Patients with Structural Epilepsy and Families

The needs of patients with structural focal epilepsy vary significant depending on the severity of epilepsy and the severity of brain damage. For many children without neurological and cognitive problems the management and parental needs are not much different than of any other type of epilepsy (see Chapter 24). However, others have also to deal not only with the epilepsy but also with the physical and mental problems caused by the brain lesions of the initial insult. These parents have difficult decisions and adaptations to make from the time that the brain damage happened and the time that epileptic seizures started. This refers to medical treatments, physical and cognitive management, educational, social and financial needs. It may be a lifelong challenge affecting many areas of life with the aim for example to help the child in achieving the maximal of its potentials.

Be prepared of what to do when an emergency occurs and seek ways of preventing them. Deep knowledge of the situation, what to expect and where to find the best medico-psycho-social and educational assistance are important.

- Get a proper assessment of the physical and mental potentials of the patient
- Some patients register in relevant websites, join support groups and share questions and answers in e-communities with other people who are going through similar problems. However you must know that not all the information you get is correct. Also the experience of one person to another may differ significantly and therefore may not apply to you

- Investigate the availability of health care (state, insurance) for the patient's health including emergency facilities. For children, regular assessment of the educational progress is needed.
- Most children should attend a mainstream school, but some of them may also need individualized education and services through the state school and health systems.
- Apart from academic progress, the child's emotional state and social adaptation should be kept under close scrutiny and any change taken seriously.
- Staff at the child's school, need to be aware of the child's condition and what to do in the event of an emergency. The school's Special Educational Needs Coordinator will usually be the person to go to about ensuring necessary arrangements and allowances are in place.

## Recommended Readings

- https://www.ncbi.nlm.nih.gov/books/NBK2605/
  This is the description of structural (symptomatic) epilepsy in the book "The epilepsies: Seizures, syndromes and management" provided by The National Center for Biotechnology Information.
- http://www.ilae.org/commission/class/diagnostic.cfm
  This is the ILAE Epilepsy Diagnosis.org which an excellent online diagnostic manual of the epilepsies, which provides information of how to diagnose seizure type(s), classify epilepsy, diagnose epilepsy syndromes and define the aetiology.

## References

1. Sillanpaa M, Schmidt D. Predicting antiepileptic drug response in children with epilepsy. Expert Rev Neurother. 2011;11:877–85.
2. Kramer G. The limitations of antiepileptic drug monotherapy. Epilepsia. 1997;38(Suppl 5):S9–S13.
3. Schmidt D. AED discontinuation may be dangerous for seizure-free patients. J Neural Transm. 2011;118:183–6.

# Women and Epilepsy

12

> *"....I made a promise to myself and to those who may suffer*
> *from any obstacle in their path that nothing would get in my*
> *way when it came to achieving what I set out to achieve... so*
> *with epilepsy in tow I've since won six world titles, two Olympic*
> *silver medals and over 180 races world wide....."*
>
> Marion Clignet

**Abstract**

Epilepsy has particularly adverse effects on girls and women in many biological and psychosocial aspects that are different from men. As a result, women with epilepsy face special challenges, especially in the area of reproductive health. The biological areas affected by epilepsy and AEDs include the menstrual cycle from menarche to menopause, sexuality and contraception, fertility, pregnancy and breastfeeding. Maternal parenting may become handicapped by safety issues due to continuing epileptic seizures and adverse drug effects. Psychosocial, safety and legal issues are also of paramount importance in women with epilepsies who take care of children, partners or parents. However, most women with epilepsy can live normal personal and family lives with determination, proper medical and psychological support and guidance, and other appropriate help.

**Keywords**

Pregnancy and epilepsy • Menstrual cycle • Sexuality and contraception • Fertility • Breastfeeding • Maternal parenting • Psychosocial • Safety and legal issues

## What Are the Fundamental Medical Differences Between Female and Male?

In medicine, the differences between male and female extend beyond the historical concept that women's health relates to reproductive hormones and organs. Certain diseases affect women exclusively, or predominantly women, and there can be

© Springer International Publishing AG 2017
T. Valeta, *The Epilepsy Book: A Companion for Patients*,
DOI 10.1007/978-3-319-61679-7_12

significant differences between the sexes in the expression of the same medical problem, and in the response to and adverse reactions to drugs. Considerations of sex and gender differences should also include psychology, behaviours and social attitudes [1, 2].

Gender-based medicine involves the study of the biological and physiological differences between the human sexes and their affect in disease. New approaches to healthcare encompass the role of sex (the classification of living things according to their reproductive hormones and organs), and the gender (a person's self-representation as male or female or how that person is responded to by social institutions on the basis of the individual's gender presentation). Such a gender-approach to health care has significant implications for medical practice. Healthcare providers need to make diagnostic and management decisions based on the sex of the patient, and respond to gender differences in how women and men approach their own health, and how they communicate their health concerns [1].

The 2001 report Exploring the Biological Contributions to Human Health: Does Sex Matter? by the Committee on Understanding the Biology of Sex and Gender Differences, Institute of Medicine explains: [3] "The study of sex differences is evolving into a mature science. There is now sufficient knowledge of the biological basis of sex differences to validate the scientific study of sex differences and to allow the generation of hypotheses with regard to health. The next step is to move from the descriptive to the experimental phase and establish the conditions that must be in place to facilitate and encourage the scientific study of the mechanisms and origins of sex differences" [3].

## Why Epilepsy Has Particular Adverse Effects on Girls and Women?

Epilepsy has particularly adverse effects on girls and women in many biological and psychosocial aspects that are different from men. As a result of these biological and social differences, women with epilepsy face special challenges, especially in the area of reproductive health.

The biological areas affected by epilepsy and AEDs include the menstrual cycle from menarche to menopause, sexuality and contraception, fertility, pregnancy and breastfeeding. Maternal parenting may become handicapped by safety issues of continuing epileptic seizures and adverse AED effects.

Psychosocial, safety and legal issues are also of paramount importance in women with epilepsies who take care of children, partners or parents.

The cultural role of women varies significantly between countries and religions. In many societies, women are mainly involved in domestic tasks and child care or enter low-paid employment out of economic necessity. In developed countries, women are more career and education oriented. These values and beliefs determine a society's attitudes towards women who have epilepsy and affect their feelings and the way they perceive themselves.

## What Are the Effects of Epilepsy in Adolescence, Puberty and Menarche?

Adolescence, puberty and menarche are associated with profound physical and psychosocial changes [5]. This transitional period from childhood to adulthood may be turbulent and often associated with a number of emotional issues.

Adolescence is a crucial period of development directed towards achieving independence and integration into society, and is associated with a variety of biological changes and emotional issues. It is marked by identity formation and self-definition, abstract thinking, experimentation with new ways of lifestyle, engaging in social activities, preparing for employment, embarking on new and intimate relationships, travelling, sleeping late and driving. Compared with their male counterparts adolescent females, experience a poorer psychosocial health in the somatic, depressive and internalizing areas [4].

Epilepsy is an additional burden for adolescents and may disturb the formation of their independence through its psychosocial, cognitive, educational and behavioural consequences, as well as the prohibition imposed by epilepsy itself on certain leisure activities, sports, employment and driving [5, 6].

Adolescents with epilepsy show significantly higher levels of depression, social anxiety, obsessive symptoms and lower competence (social competence, activity and school achievement) compared with adolescents without epilepsy [7]. Low levels of knowledge about epilepsy are significantly associated with higher levels of depression, suicidality, lower levels of self-esteem and higher levels of social anxiety. A higher intake of AEDs and concern about seizure recurrence accounts for poorer health-related quality of life.

Girls with epilepsy report more positive perceptions in the stigma and social support domains [8]. Adolescent girls are also extremely sensitive to the cosmetic adverse effects of AEDs, such as weight gain, and anorexia is often a problem.

## How Women with Epilepsy Deal with Dating and Sexual Relationships?

Emotional and sexual intimacy, timing and speed of development, extent of involvement, and amount of personal information shared with others, are influenced by many factors including age, personality, attitudes, experience, and general cultural, family and religious values. These can be areas of anxiety and may expose some individuals to physical, social and emotional risk.

Poor esteem is extremely common among girls and women with epilepsy who also have many fears about forming intimate relationships: "Shall I tell him or not?", "What if I have a seizure while with him?", "He will run away if he finds out", "I better avoid the relation so as not to get frustrated and hurt". These are realistic worries considering the attitude of people towards epilepsy. However, women with epilepsy often find the right partner and go on to have a strong and happy lifelong relationship.

The fertility and sexuality of women with epilepsy may be affected by mental, psychological and hormonal factors. Sexual activity creates more anxiety in women with epilepsy than in those without epilepsy. However, women with well-controlled epilepsy have normal sexual desire and ability to achieve orgasm though some due to medication may experience painful intercourse because of lack of lubrication and tightness due to medication.

http://www.epilepsyfoundation.org/livingwithepilepsy/gendertopics/women-shealthtopics/epilepsy-and-sexual-relationships.cfm

## What Is the Best Birth Control-Contraception of Women with Epilepsy?

Birth control (contraception) enables women to prevent unwanted pregnancies, planning and spacing their family according to their personal needs and preferences. For women with epilepsy, particularly those on AEDs, the choice of the most suitable birth control method is important.

All available birth control methods can be used by persons with epilepsy. These include:

- barriers: diaphragms, spermicidal vaginal creams, intrauterine devices (IUDs) and condoms;
- timing: the "rhythm method" where intercourse is avoided during a woman's ovulation period or withdrawal by the man prior to ejaculation;
- hormonal contraception: birth control pills, hormone implants, or hormone injections.

Of these, hormonal contraception is the most reliable method for most women, but it is not 100% effective, especially in women with epilepsy. Keep in mind that even in the general population there is always a slight chance of an unwanted pregnancy despite appropriate use of contraceptives. Antiepileptic drugs may make your hormonal birth control less reliable, resulting in an unwanted pregnancy. This is because some of the AEDs increase the breakdown of contraceptive hormones (estrogen and progesterone) in the body, making them less effective in preventing pregnancy. They are carbamazepine, oxcarbazepine, phenytoin, phenobarbital, topiramate. Valproate and levetiracetam do not interfere with the effectiveness of hormonal birth control. Lamotrigine may make the contraceptive pill slightly less effective and the pill may also make the lamotrigine less effective and increase your risk of seizures. Therefore, the doses of both medications may need to be adjusted. Discuss with your physician what the best method is for you and what adjustments in dose you may make if on AEDs and hormonal contraception.

   http://www.patient.co.uk/health/Epilepsy-Contraception-/-Preg.-Issues.htm
   http://www.epilepsy.org.uk/info/contraception
   http://www.epilepsysociety.org.uk/AboutEpilepsy/Epilepsyandyou/
Womenandepilepsy-1
   http://www.epilepsyfoundation.org/livingwithepilepsy/gendertopics/women-
shealthtopics/index.cfm
   http://www.epilepsy.com/info/women

## How Epilepsy Affects Motherhood and Parenting?

Becoming a mother and caring for your children is a splendid thing for those women who are able to become mothers. Biological mothers conceive, gestate, go into labour, give birth and can provide parenting to their child from birth until adulthood. This will ensure the physical, intellectual, and emotional security and development of the child.

Approximately one-third of people with epilepsy are women of childbearing age. All stages of motherhood present particular challenges to women with epilepsy that require significant adjustments in lifestyle in order to care for their children. However, the risks are often overemphasized and many physicians and patients consider them higher than they truly are. As a consequence women with epilepsy are often mistakenly advised to avoid becoming pregnant and/or care for their children.

The decision to become a mother and parent is personal and should be based on accurate information about the risks and how to prevent and minimize them. The type of epilepsy and type of seizures are particularly important when making this decision. There are many illustrative descriptions of women who have had successful pregnancies and healthy children contrary to advice they were given. An understanding and supportive husband/partner is however crucial.

Pregnancy, labour and the postpartum period may affect the frequency and severity of seizures and the metabolism of AEDs. The fetus may be harmed by AEDs and also by concurring convulsive seizures of the mother. Expert preconception counselling, follow- up and management during pregnancy and delivery (sometimes in specialized maternity units for epilepsy) are essential parts of good medical practice for women with epilepsy.

With proper information, guidelines and management, most women with epilepsy will have uncomplicated pregnancies and deliver normal children.

Parenting presents a number of concerns for a woman with epilepsy from the day that the child is born until adulthood. These concerns relate to the physical, emotional and social safety of the child of a mother who may have seizures when carrying out her multiple maternal duties. Mothers with active epilepsy face certain limitations to their parenting objectives, as a result of seizures that may harm them or their child, the sedative and other adverse effects of AEDs, psychological disorders and even lack of motivation. According to a report, the most problematic areas for mothers with epilepsy were caring for their baby outside the home and bathing them [9]. This also meant that some babies were put at undue risk. Breastfeeding was rated as much less problematic.

Safety advice and recommendations, most of which are common sense, can be found on many dedicated websites (see also Chap. 22 on safety in epilepsy).

The impact of parents' epilepsy on children may be profound. Disclosure of the problem by the parents may allow their children regardless their ages to adjust to the epilepsy while maintaining trust in and concern for both parents [10]. Conversely, parents concealing their epilepsy faced the most anger and resentment when the children found out about it.

## What Is the Effect of Epilepsy in Pregnancy?

Most women with epilepsy can and do have normal pregnancies providing they follow a few traditional rules for having a healthy pregnancy and child. The outlook for pregnant women with epilepsy and their offspring is excellent. The risks to mothers and their babies are small and often preventable. Overall, 95% of women with epilepsy have uncomplicated pregnancies and deliver normal babies. This rate can be significantly improved with proper management; any serious harm to the baby or mother, particularly if it is avoidable, is too much for the family that is affected.

AED treatment during pregnancy is considered necessary for most women with epilepsy, because uncontrolled maternal convulsive seizures pose a greater risk to the foetus than the use of AEDs and may also harm the mother. It is also important to remember that the concentration of AEDs may change significantly during pregnancy and the postnatal period resulting in an increase in seizures or toxicity.

It is generally accepted that AED treatment during the first three months of pregnancy is associated with a small, but significant, increase in the risk of major congenital malformations (MCM) for the baby.

- The risk of MCM in women with epilepsy who are not taking AEDs is small (probably less than twice the background rate in the general population around 1–2%)
- The risk is 3–5 times higher with valproate monotherapy and probably with topiramate,
- The risk is more than ten times in combination AEDs and particularly those with valproate and lamotrigine.
- The higher the plasma AED concentration, the higher the relative risk of MCM.

## Women Whose Children Have Epilepsy

The impact of children's epilepsy on parents is immense and extends far beyond practical issues of physical safety and the development of the child and its functioning within the family and society. As a result, parental needs are numerous, and continuous but are often unmet from the time of first diagnosis [5, 6]. Stigma has profound effects on social identity, discrimination, and overall quality of life. Facing all of these situations, parental anxiety increases and the parents themselves suffer a diminished quality of life.

The impact of children's epilepsies and the resulting parenting needs are even greater for mothers whose traditional primary role, in most societies, is raising of their children. In most Western countries since the late twentieth century, however, the role of the father in child care has been given greater prominence. In a recent study mothers sustained a greater burden of care and exhibited higher levels of strain and showed higher levels of anxiety for the future and academic achievement of their children, than fathers. Many stopped working either temporarily or indefinitely in order to care for their child.

Parents needs require more than medical therapeutic support. This is a matter of a competent healthcare system involving a multidisciplinary team, including physicians, specialist nurses, psychologists, psychotherapists and pharmacists. The community and the family should recognize the difficulties that mothers of children with epilepsy face and assist them whenever possible.

## Menopause and Elderly Women with Epilepsy

Menopause and old age are associated with significant physical and psychosocial changes. The menopause tends to occur earlier in women with epilepsy and in certain types of pre-existing epilepsy, seizure improvement or deterioration may occur. Hormone replacement therapy is not usually contraindicated.

Elderly women have an increased risk for osteoporosis and fractures.

## Personal Accounts of Women Dealing with Epilepsy

The personal accounts of women with epilepsy highlight how all the disease-related difficulties outlined above can be overcome successfully. *Epilepsy Mine*, a collection of personal accounts from women living with epilepsy, testify to its impact on women's view of themselves, their aspirations and their everyday lives.

https://www.epilepsy.org.uk/involved/campaigns/women/mine

"I now know it isn't necessarily a problem and in a way I'm grateful to epilepsy for teaching me that life should be lived and nothing should ever be taken for granted".

"We need help to achieve our goals and dreams, not simply have our concerns dismissed".

There are many great achievers among women with epilepsy and this is despite the fact that it was considerably more difficult for women to become prominent figures than it was for men. Many women with epilepsy are also professional achievers in medicine, law, the arts, and politics.

Two women Olympic medalists who have epilepsy illustrate that success may be achieved even when maximal physical strength and endurance are required.

Chanda Gunn, goalkeeper and Olympic bronze medal winner for the US Olympic women's hockey team has had juvenile absence epilepsy, which also manifested with generalized tonic-clonic seizures and photosensitivity, since 9 years of age.

Marion Clignet, Olympic cyclist, was diagnosed with epilepsy at 22 years of age. "Finding out I had epilepsy made me want to push myself harder to ensure I didn't have any excuse not to make it to the top."

In my practice I have met women who have epilepsy and who have overcome most difficulties in their lives with determination, appropriate medical and psychological support and guidance, and appropriate help. Most of these women live normal personal and family lives with few limitations.

## Recommended Readings

- http://www.epilepsyfoundation.org/living/women/index.cfm.    http://www.epilepsyontario.org/client/EO/EOWeb.nsf/0000/$seachForm?SearchView&Seq=1
- http://www.epilepsy.org.uk/info/women
- http://www.epilepsynse.org.uk/pages/info/leaflets/women.cfm
- http://www.epilepsy.com/information/women-and-epilepsy
- epilepsy in pregnancy: https://www.rcog.org.uk/globalassets/documents/guidelines/green-top-guidelines/gtg68_epilepsy.pdf

## References

1. Pinn VW. Sex and gender factors in medical studies: implications for health and clinical practice. JAMA. 2003;289:397–400.
2. Butler J. Bodies that matter: on the discursive limits of sex. New York: Routledge; 2001.
3. Committee on Understanding the Biology of Sex and Gender Differences BoHSP. Exploring the biological contributions to human health: does sex matter? Washington, DC: National Academy Press; 2001.
4. Raty LK, Larsson G, Soderfeldt BA, Larsson BM. Psychosocial aspects of health in adolescence: the influence of gender, and general self-concept. J Adolesc Health. 2005;36:530.
5. Valeta T. Impact of epilepsies on women and related psychosocial issues. In: Panayiotopoulos CP, Crawford P, Tomson T, editors. Epilepsies in girls and women, vol. 4. Oxford: Medicinae; 2008. p. 190–7.
6. Valeta T, Sogawa Y, Moshe SL. Impact of focal seizures on patients and family. In: Panayiotopoulos CP, Benbadis S, Sisodiya S, editors. Focal epilepsies: seizures, syndromes and management, vol. 5. Oxford: Medicinae; 2008. p. 230–8.
7. Baker GA, Spector S, McGrath Y, Soteriou H. Impact of epilepsy in adolescence: a UK controlled study. Epilepsy Behav. 2005;6:556–62.
8. Stevanovic D. Health-related quality of life in adolescents with well-controlled epilepsy. Epilepsy Behav. 2007;10:571–5.
9. Bagshaw J, Crawford P, Chappell B. Problems that mothers' with epilepsy experience when caring for their children. Seizure. 2008;17:42–8.
10. Lechtenberg R, Akner L. Psychologic adaptation of children to epilepsy in a parent. Epilepsia. 1984;25:40–5.

# Mortality and Sudden Unexpected Death in Epilepsy (SUDEP)

**13**

**Abstract**

Epilepsy is associated with an increased risk of death, 2–3 greater than in the general population. This excess is mainly related to associated or underlying disease that has caused epilepsy (structural lesions, infections, tumours), accidents and drowning because of seizures, and convulsive status epilepticus. Sudden unexpected death in epilepsy (SUDEP) is a less common reason for the increased mortality in epilepsy and may be the result of the direct effect of an epileptic (usually convulsive) seizure on the cardiorespiratory (heart and lungs) system or the brain itself. Most cases of SUDEP involve young patients (from late teens to late forties) with a long history of tonic-clonic seizures. Frequently SUDEP occurs in sleep. In many patients antiepileptic drug levels are generally low.

**Keywords**

Epilepsy bereaved • SUDEP aware • Standardised mortality ratio • Tonic clonic seizures • Nontraumatic death • Nondrowning death

## Are People with Epilepsy at Increased Risk for Death?

Research has shown that epilepsy is associated with an increased risk of death (mortality) [1–4]. The number of deaths in a population with epilepsy is two to three times greater than that in the general population. This excess is mainly related to associated or underlying disease and less often directly attributable to epilepsy as in sudden unexpected death (SUDEP). Death from epilepsy is uncommon in children with no neurological disorder. In addition, in children, SUDEP is rare [5].

© Springer International Publishing AG 2017
T. Valeta, *The Epilepsy Book: A Companion for Patients*,
DOI 10.1007/978-3-319-61679-7_13

## What Is the Cause of Death in Epilepsy?

Death in epilepsy is mainly due to the underlying disease in the brain that has caused epilepsy (structural lesions, infections, tumours), accidents and drowning because of seizures, and convulsive status epilepticus. This premature death is most likely to happen in people with severe epilepsy, frequent epileptic seizures, neurological abnormalities, erroneous treatments and non-compliance.

Patients with epilepsy may die because of accident secondary to a seizure or as a consequence of a seizure. Drowning remains a common cause of death. Patients with epilepsy and psychiatric comorbidities have a higher risk of suicide. Convulsive status epilepticus has a high degree of mortality, probably reaching 37%. Some serious adverse reactions of antiepileptic drugs may be fatal.

Sudden unexpected death in epilepsy is a less common reason for the increased mortality in epilepsy and may be the result of the direct effect of an epileptic (usually convulsive) seizure on the cardiorespiratory (heart and lungs) system or the brain itself.

SUDEP is the term used for nontraumatic and nondrowning death which occurs without warning in a person and where the post-mortem (autopsy) fails to establish any other cause of death [6]. Most cases involve young patients (from late teens to late forties) with a long history of tonic-clonic seizures. Frequently the patients are found dead in bed. In many patients antiepileptic drug serum levels are generally sub-therapeutic. There may be a genetically determined burden to SUDEP for a few people with epilepsy.

SUDEP is more common in patients

- between ages 20 and 40 years.
- with uncontrolled and frequent predominantly convulsive seizures (mainly those occurring in sleep).
- with many years of seizures (most persons who die of SUDEP have had epilepsy for 15–20 years).
- with early than late onset epilepsy.
- with concurrent disorders-particularly severe learning difficulties and developmental disabilities
- on multiple antiepileptic treatments (but this may indicate the severity of epilepsy)
- while asleep in bed

## Should the Possibility of Death in Epilepsy Revealed to Patients and Relatives?

The possibility of death during a seizure is of concern to patients and parents and may be already in their mind before medical consultation. Therefore this question may arise by them during the consultation.

The question of whether and when to discuss SUDEP with patients and families has been vigorously debated in recent years. Those against it, argue that this may cause undue distress, the risks are low, the mechanisms are not well understood and prevention is uncertain. Others argue that this should be discussed selectively only for patients of severe epilepsy or those with poor compliance to treatment. At the other end, including patients' advocates such as Epilepsy Bereaved in the UK, believe that patients with epilepsy, as with any other condition, have the right to know the risks associated with their diagnosis and this is a legal obligation of physicians. A physician might be legally liable in the event of death for not having discussed this issue with the patient.

## How Death in Epilepsy Can Be Prevented?

This can be achieved by minimizing the risk factors for death such as improving control of seizures with appropriate management, compliance, safety care and avoidance of accidents. In regard to prevention of SUDEP though this is uncertain, advice may be given for those with convulsive seizures on preferring the supine (and not the prone) position in sleep, supervision, regular checks or use of a listening device in sleep, compliance with proper medication [7]. Various home seizure detection systems have been marketed, including pulse oximetry, heart rate monitors, bed motion monitors, and accelerometers. However: a. the ability of these monitors to reliably detect seizures remains problematic, and in many cases, frequent false positive alarms have limited their use and b. even prompt cardiovascular resuscitation by medical personnel may be inadequate to prevent SUDEP in some cases.

## Formal Recommendations About SUDEP

The 2012 National Institute of Clinical Excellence (NICE) recommendations on SUDEP are:

- Information on SUDEP should be included in literature on epilepsy to show why preventing seizures is important.
- Tailored information on the person's relative risk of SUDEP should be part of the counselling checklist for children, young people and adults with epilepsy and their families and/or carers.
- The risk of SUDEP can be minimised by optimising seizure control and being aware of the potential consequences of nocturnal seizures.
- Tailored information and discussion between the child, young person or adult with epilepsy, their family and/or carers (as appropriate) and healthcare professionals should take account of the small but definite risk of SUDEP.
- Where families and/or carers have been affected by SUDEP, healthcare professionals should contact families and/or carers to offer their condolences, invite them to discuss the death, and offer referral to bereavement counselling and a SUDEP support group.

See: Diagnosis and Management of the Epilepsies in Children: www.nice.org.uk/pdf/cg020childrenquickrefguide.pdf

## Recommendations to Patients with Epilepsy and Their Family

It should be remember that although death from epilepsy is a realistic possibility this is small and it is unlikely to happen in otherwise normal patients and particularly those without convulsive seizures and well controlled epilepsy. It is fully legitimate to discuss these matters with your health care professionals but first make yourself aware of whether you or your child have any of the risks factors connected with the possibility of death in epilepsy through reading of this chapter and from the recommended interned sites (see below). In addition to other appropriate tests, an electrocardiogram should be requested for all patients with epilepsy.

## Recommended Readings

- SUDEP: continuing the Global Conversation deals with epilepsy-related death and covers the impact of epilepsy-related death and its burden from the public health perspective.
  http://www.sudepglobalconversation.com/page/contents.html
- Partners Against Mortality in Epilepsy (PAME)
  http://www.aesnet.org/pame/
- Epilepsy bereaved or SUDEP action
  http://www.sudep.org/
- SUDEP Aware
  http://www.sudepaware.org/
- For judicial cases of SUDEP, recommendations and parents reactions see:
  http://www.sudep.org/whatwedo/investigatory-reports-on-epilepsy-deaths/fatal-accident-inquiry-into-the-deaths-of-erin-casey-and-christina-ilia/)
- For the tragic accounts of people who lost a loved one to SUDEP see http://www.sudep.org/forum/viewforum.php?f=3

## References

1. Levira F, Thurman DJ, Sander JW, Hauser WA, Hesdorffer DC, Masanja H, et al. Premature mortality of epilepsy in low- and middle-income countries: a systematic review from the Mortality Task Force of the International League Against Epilepsy. Epilepsia. 2017;58:6–16.
2. Thurman DJ, Logroscino G, Beghi E, Hauser WA, Hesdorffer DC, Newton CR, et al. The burden of premature mortality of epilepsy in high-income countries: a systematic review from the Mortality Task Force of the International League Against Epilepsy. Epilepsia. 2017;58:17–26.
3. Jallon P. Mortality in patients with epilepsy. Curr Opin Neurol. 2004;17:141–6.
4. Forsgren L, Hauser WA, Olafsson E, Sander JW, Sillanpaa M, Tomson T. Mortality of epilepsy in developed countries: a review. Epilepsia. 2005;46(Suppl 11):18–27.
5. Camfield P, Camfield C. Sudden unexpected death in people with epilepsy: a pediatric perspective. Semin Pediatr Neurol. 2005;12:10–4.

6. Nashef L, So EL, Ryvlin P, Tomson T. Unifying the definitions of sudden unexpected death in epilepsy. Epilepsia. 2012;53:227–33.
7. Ryvlin P, Nashef L, Tomson T. Prevention of sudden unexpected death in epilepsy: a realistic goal? Epilepsia. 2013;54(Suppl 2):23–8.

# Investigations for Epileptic Seizures

**14**

**Abstract**

The diagnosis of epilepsy is mainly based on the clinical information. However, a number of investigations (laboratory procedures) may be requested in order to make certain that the diagnosis is correct. The main laboratory procedures for a patient with possible or definite epileptic seizures are the electroencephalogram (EEG) and the brain imaging (brain MRI and brain CT scan). A physician may also request blood and urine test, ECG (electrocardiograph) or even more specific investigations such as metabolic or toxicology screening and molecular genetic testing. These depend on the particular clinical problem and individual patient.

**Keywords**

Electroencephalogram • Video-EEG • EEG telemetry • Brain imaging • Brain magnetic imaging • Computerized axial tomography • Genetic testing

## What Are the Main Investigations for the Diagnosis of Epilepsy?

The diagnosis of epilepsy is mainly based on the clinical information [1]. However, a number of investigations (laboratory procedures) may be requested in order to make certain that the diagnosis is correct, find out its cause and shape the proper management. The results of these tests are added to the other information and provide a clearer picture of what is wrong in that particular person.

The main laboratory procedures for a patient with possible or definite epileptic seizures are the:

- electroencephalogram (EEG) and the
- brain imaging (brain MRI and brain CT scan)

© Springer International Publishing AG 2017
T. Valeta, *The Epilepsy Book: A Companion for Patients*,
DOI 10.1007/978-3-319-61679-7_14

These tests are usually done by technologists and assessed by a specialist physician. The results from the tests are then passed back to the doctor in charge of the patient for proper evaluation.

However, a physician may also request blood and urine test, ECG (electrocardiograph) or even more specific investigations such as metabolic or toxicology screening and molecular genetic testing. These depend on the particular clinical problem and individual patient. Their aim is to provide definite diagnosis of a specific disorder. Genetic testing has become available for a growing number of hereditary disorders associated with epileptic seizures.

Investigative procedures are more demanding in children than in adults, or in those in whom seizures are amongst the first symptoms of a disease than in those where the main disease has already been established.

## Electroencephalography (EEG)

The EEG is the most important test in the diagnosis and management of epilepsies [1–4]. It was invented in 1923 by the German Hans Berger and it is harmless and relatively inexpensive. It records the electrical activity of the brain through surface electrodes placed on the scalp similar to electrocardiography which records the cardiac electrical rhythms through electrodes placed on the chest.

The role of the EEG is to help the physician establish an accurate diagnosis. It is indispensable in the correct diagnosis of the type of epileptic seizure or syndrome. In this sense, it is mandatory for all patients with epileptic seizures to have at least an EEG even after a single seizure.

However, there are many problems for the correct interpretation of the EEG and this may lead to serious diagnostic errors. The EEG should always be assessed according to the individual patient's personal history.

## Is the EEG Specific for Epilepsy?

In many epileptic conditions, the EEG may confirm the correct diagnosis. In others, it may not be helpful because the EEG may be consistently normal in a significant number of patients with epilepsy or abnormal in non-epileptic patients.

However, for the EEG to provide accurate assessments, it must be properly performed by experienced technologists and carefully studied and interpreted in the context of a well-described clinical setting by experienced physicians. Otherwise, it may be misleading and result in serious diagnostic errors. A request for an EEG should describe the clinical problem well, and the EEG technologist should also obtain and supplement the relevant clinical information.

Patients with epilepsy frequently have focal or generalized paroxysmal EEG abnormalities even at times that they do not have seizures.

An EEG in patients with chronic epilepsies or those who are on appropriate anti-epileptic drug (AED) medication may be uninformative or misleading. Obtaining previous medical and EEG reports is essential.

Certain factors or conditions may interfere with the EEG activity such as low blood sugar (hypoglycemia) caused by fasting, drugs and mainly neuroleptics and sedatives.

Ambulatory EEG and video EEG telemetry is used when diagnosis is proving difficult to identify seizure type or other non-epileptic paroxysmal attacks.

## Principles of EEG

The brain electrical activity is picked up by electrodes (small metallic disks or pads) attached to the scalp. These are connected to the EEG machine, which detects and amplifies the electrical signals and records them in paper (old analog EEG) though today the EEG is displayed and viewed on computer screens (digital recordings).

## How the EEG Is Performed?

The test is performed by an EEG technologist. First the technologist will measure the head so that the electrodes can be placed in the correct position. A wax crayon, which can be easily washed off later, is used to mark the points on the scalp where the electrodes should be placed. The technologist will probably scrub each position on the scalp with a mildly abrasive cream before applying the electrodes. This will help improve the quality of the recording. Usually the electrodes are held in place by a paste that can be washed off easily when the test is over.

After the EEG recording is done, the technologist will remove the electrodes, wash the paste out of the hair and the patient can go home.

The EEG report is done by qualified physicians after studying the electrical traces on the computer screen or paper.

These arrangements, and the way tests are performed, may vary between different EEG departments.

## Preparing Yourself for an EEG

Wash your hair the night before using only shampoo and water. Do not use styling aids such as hair gels, mousse, hairspray or oils of any kind. These products can interfere with the electrodes and limit the usefulness of the test.

Eat normally and take your regularly scheduled medications.

## Risks of the EEG

The EEG test is painless, harmless and causes no discomfort. The electrodes only pick up electrical activity they don't give out electrical signals or any sensations that is the EEG does not affect the brain.

However, a seizure, usually minor, may be provoked by certain activating techniques such as overbreathing, intermittent photic stimulation and sleep deprivation which are often desirable for diagnostic reasons.

Some patients may also experience faints usually at the time of placing the electrodes. Skin irritation or redness may be present at the locations where the electrodes were placed, but this will wear off in a few hours.

## Routine EEG

This is usually performed at an outpatient's appointment at the hospital. The entire procedure takes about 1 h which includes 20–30 min for the preparation and 20–40 for the actual EEG recording. Medication should not be stopped for the test unless otherwise advised by the treating physician. The patient goes home as soon as the test has been done.

The recording takes place in a quiet, often dimly lit, room while the patient is sitting still in a chair or lie on a couch (movements can affect the quality of the recording and affect its interpretation). The patient is asked to close and open his/her eyes at certain intervals because these are associated with different EEG patterns.

A routine EEG also includes two activation procedures (1) hyperventilation (deep breathing) for 2.5–3 min and (2) intermittent photic stimulation (flickering stroboscopic light). These can sometimes trigger patterns of electrical activity in the brain which are associated with certain types of epilepsy. During the recording the patient may fall asleep which is often desirable. An EEG during sleep may provide useful information (see EEG after sleep deprivation).

## Video-EEG

Most of the modern EEGs machines video tape the patient simultaneously with the EEG. Thus when a seizure occurs, the video EEG correlates step by step the clinical symptoms with the electrical discharges (ictal EEG). The video image and the EEG can be viewed together on a split-screen display, with the EEG on one side and the video image on the other, or separate monitors can be used for the two sets of information.

## Sleep EEG Tests

An EEG in drowsiness, sleep and awakening is important for the purposes of increasing the chance of detecting specific brain activity and improve diagnosis. It is particularly useful in patients who produce a normal routine awake EEG or in those whose seizures consistently occur during sleep and/or after awakening from sleep. It is done in the same way as the routine EEG but while the patients is asleep.

To achieve sleep for the purpose of obtaining an EEG during sleep, EEG departments have different practices:

- sleep deprivation (partial or all night)
- drug-induced sleep.

The best practice is to perform a sleep EEG that is as close as possible to the natural state and habits of the patient, and thereby achieve best results with minimal risk to the patient and minimal discomfort to the patient and their family.

## Ambulatory EEG Tests

An ambulatory EEG records the brain electrical activity throughout the daily life of the patients (day and night), over a period of one or more, usually 3–4 days. The patient carries out his/her normal activities while the recordings are being made. The test is harmless and painless. Its main purpose is to make long recordings and particularly to find out whether the habitual attacks of the patient are associated with electrical seizure abnormalities and their types.

## Video EEG Telemetry

This is like a video-EEG performed over 5–7 days in a hospital ward or specialised video-telemetry unit. Its purpose is to record the attacks of the patient in order to make sure that these are epileptic seizures and/or to determine their onset in the brain if neurosurgery is considered. It can also rule out other conditions that might be causing the attacks such as psychogenic or cardiogenic fits.

Patients receive detail information of what video EEG telemetry involves, what to do and what not to do during their stay in the hospital.

## Brain Imaging in Epilepsy

Brain imaging is performed to help find the cause of seizures by producing pictures of the brain (structure of the brain) which might show abnormal areas such as scarring, tumors, infections, atrophy, strokes, malformations of the brain, and abnormal blood vessels that may be responsible for epileptic seizures [1, 5]. The two common types of brain scan are:

• Magnetic Resonance Imaging (MRI) and
• Computerised Axial Tomography (CT).

Both produce pictures of how the brain looks. The MRI is superior to CT scan in finding even minor lesions.

Brain imaging may not be needed for patients with definite idiopathic epilepsies such as rolandic epilepsy, juvenile myoclonic epilepsy and childhood absence epilepsy because the results are expected to be normal.

## Are There Any Risks from Brain Imaging

Both CT and MRI are painless and relatively safe. However, radiation is used in CT scans and therefore pregnant women are offered other methods of testing that do not impose risk to the foetus. The MRI does not involve exposing the body to radiation and there is no evidence that there is a risk from the magnetic and radio waves that are used in MRI.

## Magnetic Resonance Imaging and Epilepsy

MRI scans are extremely helpful in looking at structural causes of epilepsy. An MRI scan uses strong magnetic fields to produce very clear pictures of the brain and any abnormality that might be causing epilepsy.

During the scan, the patient need to lie still inside a narrow tube, which is confining and can upset people who don't like enclosed spaces. The machine also makes clicking and buzzing noises. Most places provide headphones with music to block this noise out.

## Other Uses of MRI

The type of MRI technique described above is used for structural imaging—that is creating an image of the brain to see how it is made up. Structural imaging is used to look for the cause of someone's epilepsy. But different MRI techniques have many other uses, showing us how our brains work and what functions or activities each area of the brain is responsible for.

## For Detail Information About MRI See:

http://www.radiologyinfo.org/en/info.cfm?pg=headmr
https://www.epilepsysociety.org.uk/closer-look-mri#.Vzsfh5ErLIU
http://www.nhs.uk/Conditions/MRI-scan/Pages/Introduction.aspx
http://fmri.ucsd.edu/Research/whatisfmri.html

## Computerised Axial Tomography (CT)

CT scans use X-rays to take images of the brain. CT scans are not suitable if you are pregnant because the X-rays could affect an unborn baby. During a CT scan the patient lies still on a couch which slides into the scanner.

CT examinations are generally painless, fast and easy. The amount of time that the patient needs to lie still is brief; 10–20 min. After the CT scan you can return to your normal activities.

Images from a CT scan are less detailed than those from MRI scans. Unlike MRI scanners, CT scanners do not make a loud noise.

## For Detail Information About CT Scans See:

http://www.radiologyinfo.org/en/info.cfm?pg=headct
http://www.nhs.uk/Conditions/CT-scan/Pages/Introduction.aspx

## Genetic Testing

There is tremendous recent progress in the genetics of epilepsy. Genetic testing is playing a significant role in clinical epilepsy practice and particularly for people with epileptic encephalopathies such as Dravet syndrome. Which patients needs genetic testings depends in part on the symptoms and age of the patient, the severity of the epilepsy but also on the desires of the family to use the information for family planning. Accurate risk information can be extremely valuable for young families. This genetic information may give people with epilepsy and their families more detail about their specific epilepsy syndrome.

## How Is Genetic Testing Done in People with Epilepsy?

Usually, genetic testing requires a blood or saliva sample to be taken from the person with epilepsy. The sample is then sent to a laboratory for genetic testing. The test looks at the DNA in the person's blood or saliva. The sample is analyzed for mutations (changes of the gene structure) in genes that have a known association with different types of epilepsy.

## How Can Genetic Testing Help People with Epilepsy, Their Families and Their Health Care Team?

- Genetic testing in a person with epilepsy can confirm a specific diagnosis and provide evidence for selecting an appropriate treatment.
- Genetic information may help to limit unnecessary or invasive investigations.
- Genetic testing provides a basis for further genetic counseling for families.

## Recommended Readings

- Genetics of the epilepsies by S. Sisodiya in: https://www.epilepsysociety.org.uk/sites/default/files/attachments/Chapter05Sisodiya2015.pdf
- Clinical Genetic Testing in Epilepsy by H. C. Mefford in: https://www.ncbi.nlm.nih.gov/pmc/articles/PMC4532232/
- Genetic Testing in Epilepsy: What Should You Be Doing? by I. E. Scheffer in: https://www.ncbi.nlm.nih.gov/pmc/articles/PMC3152152/
- Epilepsy Foundation in: http://www.epilepsy.com/learn/diagnosis/genetic-testing.

## References

1. Panayiotopoulos CP. The epilepsies: seizures, syndromes and management. Oxford: Bladon Medical Publishing; 2005. https://www.ncbi.nlm.nih.gov/books/NBK2601/
2. Binnie CD, Stefan H. Modern electroencephalography: its role in epilepsy management. Clin Neurophysiol. 1999;110:1671–97.
3. Herman ST, Takeoka M, Hughes JR, Drislane FW. Electroencephalography in clinical epilepsy research. Epilepsy Behav. 2011;22:126–33.
4. Leach JP, Stephen LJ, Salveta C, Brodie MJ. Which electroencephalography (EEG) for epilepsy? The relative usefulness of different EEG protocols in patients with possible epilepsy. J Neurol Neurosurg Psychiatry. 2006;77:1040–2.
5. Duncan JS, Winston GP, Koepp MJ, Ourselin S. Brain imaging in the assessment for epilepsy surgery. Lancet Neurol. 2016;15:420–33.

# Prophylactic Treatment with Antiepileptic Drugs (AED)

# 15

**Abstract**

The main treatment of epilepsy is usually with antiepileptic drugs taken daily for as long as the patient has active epilepsy (prophylactic treatment). The aim of treatment is total freedom or maximal reduction of seizures and best quality of life without significant side effects. Currently, there are 9 "old AEDs" and 17 "new AEDs". Each of these AEDs, old or new, serves its own purpose, has specific efficacy in certain types of epileptic seizures, side effects, and interactions. AED, like any other drug, are associated with side effects. These may be mild and short-lived but others may be severe. Side effects of AEDs should be thoroughly sought and assessed in treated patients. Approximately, 70–80% of patients respond well to a single (monotherapy) or combined drug (polytherapy) prophylactic treatment.

**Keywords**

Monotherapy • Polytherapy • Seizure-freedom • Side effects • Adverse drug reactions • Drug interactions • Generic drug name • Brand drug name • Titration

## What Is the Prophylactic Treatment with Antiepileptic Drugs?

The main treatment of epilepsy is usually with antiepileptic drugs (Table 15.1) taken daily for as long as the patient has active epilepsy (prophylactic treatment) [1–9]. Monotherapy is when only one AED is used. Polytherapy is when two or more AEDs are used. Polytherapy should be avoided if possible mainly because drugs may interfere one the other resulting in therapeutic failures and increased side effects. However, polytherapy is needed for 30–50% of patients whose seizures are not controlled with one drug. In one fifth of patients, AEDs are ineffective and these patients are candidates either for neurosurgical interventions or other non-pharmacological treatments.

**Table 15.1**  Available
antiepileptic drugs

| Nine "old AEDs" from 1912 to 1989 |
| --- |
| • Phenobarbitone 1912 |
| • Phenytoin 1938 |
| • Primidone 1952 |
| • Ethosuximide 1955 |
| • Sulthiame 1960 |
| • Carbamazapine 1965 |
| • Sodium Valproate 1973 |
| • Clonazepam 1974 |
| • Clobazam 1979 |
| Seventeen "new AEDs" have been introduced in clinical practice after 1989: |
| • Vigabatrin 1989 |
| • Lamotrigine 1991 |
| • Felbamate 1993 |
| • Gabapentin 1993 |
| • Piracetam 1993 |
| • Topiramate 1995 |
| • Tiagabine 1998 |
| • Oxcarbazepine 2000 |
| • Levetiracetam 2000 |
| • Pregabalin 2004 |
| • Zonisamide 2005 |
| • Rufinamide 2007 |
| • Eslicarbazepine 2009 |
| • Lacosamide 2009 |
| • Stiripentol 2011 |
| • Retigabine 2011 |
| • Perampanel 2014 |
| • Brivaracetam 2016 |

## What Is the Aim of AED Treatment in Epilepsy?

The aim of treatment in epilepsy is:

- total freedom or maximal reduction of seizures and particularly the severe ones
- no significant side effects from drugs
- best quality of life with regard to physical, mental, educational, social and psychological functioning of the patient

A requirement for any treatment is that the patient truly suffers from epileptic seizures. Do not forget that a quarter of patients treated for 'epilepsy' do not suffer genuine epileptic seizures (see psychogenic nonepileptic seizures, Chapter 17).

Correct diagnosis is a must for the success of therapeutic decisions because the choice of AED depends on seizure type.

The treatment goal cannot be achieved satisfactorily without a thorough evaluation of the patient's seizures, medical history, possible co medication for other diseases and the individual patient's circumstances. Patients and parents should be well informed about the purpose of AED medication, and its efficacy, side effects and possible length of treatment.

Special groups of patients with epileptic disorders require particular attention and management. Children, elderly people, women (particularly of childbearing age) and patients with mental, physical and other comorbidities are vulnerable and their treatment is more demanding.

## Old and New AEDs

There is a tendency and you may get confused with the use of terms such as old and new AEDs (Table 15.1). In our days, there are numerous messages and articles portraying the benefits of new versus the old AEDs. Therefore, it is very reasonable to ask the question whether the new drugs offer a significant benefit.

Nine "old AEDs" that have been used for many years in the treatment of epilepsy and seventeen "new AEDs" introduced in clinical practice after 1989 are listed in Table 15.1. Each of these AEDs, old or new, serves its own purpose, has specific efficacy in certain types of epileptic seizures, side effects, and interactions.

Generally there is a substantiated view that the new AEDs are as good as the old ones in controlling epilepsy but they are better tolerated with less side effects and less interactions with other drugs.

Patients should discuss the relative advantages and disadvantages of different drug choices with an informed physician.

## What Is the Cost of Treatment with AEDs?

Cost of treatment should not be an issue in medicine, but in reality this is a major factor of concern particularly in resource poor countries and when medication is not freely provided by national health systems or personal health insurance. All newer AEDs are very expensive in relation to older generation AEDs.

## What Are the Side Effects of AEDs?

Any drug is associated with side effects (adverse drug reactions). Even the most innocent over-the-counter drugs like aspirin or paracetamol can have serious side effects that may be lethal for a few patients. The same is true for AEDs.

Side effects of AEDs should be thoroughly sought and assessed in treated patients.

Despite their significance, their detection is often neglected because:

- Patients may be reluctant or be embarrassed to report them: they may confuse them with a consequence of their illness or they may accept them as unavoidable in order to achieve seizure freedom (a price to pay)
- Some of them may be inconspicuous or become apparent after many years of AED use
- Physicians may not ask for them because of time constraints or may misinterpret them as symptoms unrelated to the treatment

AED side effects may be minor or severe, transient or progressive, reversible or irreversible, acute or chronic, known, unknown or suspected. They vary significantly between AEDs and with dose, length of exposure, individual susceptibility, age, sex and comorbitidies. Side effects are more likely to occur with polytherapy than monotherapy.

Patients, particularly with newly identified epilepsy, are susceptible to develop side effects. Some patients develop side effects easily even with small AED doses while others are resistant to side effects even at the maximum doses.

## Life-Threatening Side Effects

These are the most dreadful of all side effects

- Hypersensitivity to AEDs syndrome is a rare but sometimes fatal side effect of AEDs. This starts with skin rash usually at the start of treatment (within days or weeks). The treating physician should be immediately informed and the drug should be stopped and replaced by another appropriate AED.
- Liver or pancreas failure particularly in infants
- Blood effects
- Cardiac effects particularly in the elderly
- Suicidal thoughts

## How to Recognise and Probably Prevent Side Effects?

When prescribed an AED, get as much information as possible from the physician and supplement this with appropriate reading. Write down and inform your physician of NEW symptoms that you noted after starting an AED and how these develop. These may be physical symptoms such as rash, easy bruising, fatigue, mental symptoms such as insomnia or drowsiness, lack of concentration, depression, sexual decline. However, remember that pharmas are listing down all possible and reported side effects even if they are not fully established thus avoiding any possible legal implications.

## What Is the Titration, Dose and Frequency of Administration of an AED?

For an AED to be effective in controlling seizures, it has to be in the blood at sufficient amounts (therapeutic range). Most of the AEDS are taken in divided doses twice a day but for others one dose per day may be sufficient. Others should be taken three times per day. AEDs that need dosing more than twice a day are not practical for patient use and may reduce compliance.

When starting with an AED, it is recommended that the full dose (this is called maintenance dose) is reached at steps of low dose and slow administration (this is called titration). The rate of titration varies amongst drugs significantly. Some need starting with a very low dose and a very slow pace of increasing the drug over time. This is to avoid side effects and prevent those that may be significant or serious.

The physician should

- Explain and give in writing the recommended dose to be used and the rate of increasing the dose of the AED.
- Warn that any type of hypersensitive reactions such as rash (even if mild) should be reported immediately so as to prevent more serious and sometimes life-threatening events.
- Clarify that minor side effects such as fatigue or drowsiness are usually dose related.

## Generic Vs. Brand AED

Generic AEDs contain the active substance of the drug. Brand AED is the name given by the pharmaceutical company when an AEDs is first licensed. For example Tegretol is the brand name of carbamazepine which is its generic name. Generic drugs are usually introduced after patents have been expired with the single aim to reduce the cost of the medication.

It is important that a patient should remain in the same brand or the particular generic product over the whole time of treatment because changing this may result in deterioration of seizures and/or increased side effects. Discuss this with your physician or pharmacist when you get your medication.

## When AED Treatment Should Be Withdrawn? Total AED Withdrawal

Consideration of total withdrawal of AEDs is needed in the following patients:

- patients who do not suffer from epileptic seizures
- patients suffering from self-limited epileptic syndromes who have reached the age of remission (see rolandic epilepsy and Panayiotopoulos syndrome)

- patients who are seizure free for more than 3–5 years, provided that they do not suffer from epileptic syndromes requiring longer treatment such as juvenile myoclonic epilepsy

Discontinuation of AEDs should be extremely slow, in small doses and in long steps of weeks or months. Before starting AED withdrawal, there is a need for a thorough reevaluation of the patient. The presence of even minor seizures indicates the need for continuation of AED treatment.

## What Is AED Monitoring and When Should This Be Performed?

Your doctor may want to know the amount of the AED in your body.
    The reason is in order to:

- best regulate your medication so as to achieve the best control of the seizures with minimal side effects or
- make sure that you take your medication correctly, or
- in pregnancy.

This is done through blood (and sometimes saliva) samples. In practice, for each AED there is a range (minimal and maximal) that most patients achieve the desired therapeutic effect with no significant side effects. This is called reference, target or therapeutic range [10].
    Repeating AED monitoring in patients who are controlled and with no signs of adverse reactions 'just to make sure that everything is ok' is often unnecessary.

## How Not to Miss or Forget Taking Your Medication?

The commonest reason for relapse of seizures in an otherwise well controlled patient is sudden discontinuation of AED treatment. This often happens when the patient forgets taking his/her drugs, misses some of them, runs out of supplies, deliberately stops taking them or misunderstands the medical instructions.
    Even the most compliant person, may miss or forget taking his medication. "Did I take it or not"? is a usual question. Therefore, it is important that patients use pill boxes (dosettes, pill organisers) which come in various shapes and forms usually for weekly (7 day) intake.
    **Dosette boxes (pill organizers, calendar blister packs)** are individualized box containing medications organised into compartments by day and time, so as to simplify the taking of medications, especially in patients with polypharmacy.
    Ask your chemist what is the best dosette box for you and to set up your prescriptions within it. This may help with any difficulty that you might have which medications to take and when.

The medication should be store in a safe and easily accessed place but out of reach for children and mentally unstable.

## Recommendations to Patients with Epilepsy and Their Family

Make sure that you have discussed with your health care professionals and understood well

- The diagnosis, seizure type, syndrome and likely prognosis
- The benefits and risks of the proposed AED treatment
- How to start and continue with your AED
- Your lifestyle and personal preferences, which must be considered when deciding the best drug for you.
- Individual risks of epilepsy, living with seizures and prevention of accidents.
- Your care plan that explains what other options are available if the first drug does not stop the seizures.

## Remember

- There are no good or bad AEDS. An AED that may be good for one patient may be bad for another one. A good AED is the one which controls epileptic seizures with no significant side effects. A bad drug is the one which may cause worsening of seizures and/or intolerable side effects.
- An AED that may be good (beneficial) for one type of epileptic seizures may be bad for another type of seizures.
- An AED may be very effective in controlling the epileptic seizures but side effects may be severe needing its replacement.
- Not all patients with epileptic seizures are in need of AEDS and often discontinuation of AEDs should be considered
- Not all physicians are familiar with AEDs, their efficacy and side effects.

Considering all these and the number of available AEDs (Table 15.1) it is important that a patient and family get the maximal and best information themselves through appropriate reading and consultation.

## Recommended Readings

- Information for any AED can be found in most websites and resources provided in Chap. 26. See for example AEDS available in the United Kingdom at http://www.epilepsy.org.uk/info/treatment/uk-anti-epileptic-drugs-list and USA at http://www.epilepsy.com/EPILEPSY/seizure_MEDICINES For other countries and languages ask your physician and the local pharmaceutical companies.

- However, the most reliable source for information (mainly for health care professionals) is obtained from the so-called 'package insert' (in the USA) and the 'summary of product characteristics' (in the EU). The package insert can be obtained from http://dailymed.nlm. Nih.gov/dailymed/about.cfm. The summary of product characteristics can be obtained in any European language from http://www.ema.europa.eu/ema/index.jsp?curl=/pages/medicines/landing/epar_search.jsp&murl=menus/medicines/medicines.jsp&mid=WC0b01ac058001d125 In UK these are also available from http://emc. Medicines.org.uk
- The ILAE provides a Worldwide AED Database at http://www.ilae.org/visitors/centre/aeds/index.cfm but this may not be updated.
- Other reliable sources of relevant information of AEDs
- http://www.epilepsysociety.org.uk/list-anti-epileptic-drugs#.VsdaovKLTIU
- https://www.epilepsy.org.uk/info/treatment/uk-anti-epileptic-drugs-list
- http://pathways.nice.org.uk/pathways/epilepsy/treating-epilepsy-with-anti-epileptic-drugs-aeds
- http://www.epilepsy.com/learn/treating-seizures-and-epilepsy/seizure-and-epilepsy-medicines/seizure-medication-list

## References

1. Rosati A, De MS, Guerrini R. Antiepileptic drug treatment in children with epilepsy. CNS Drugs. 2015;29:847–63.
2. Perucca E, Tomson T. The pharmacological treatment of epilepsy in adults. Lancet Neurol. 2011;10:446–56.
3. Asconape JJ. The selection of antiepileptic drugs for the treatment of epilepsy in children and adults. Neurol Clin. 2010;28:843–52.
4. Beghi E, DiFrancesco JC. Treatment of drug resistant epilepsy. In: Panayiotopoulos CP, editor. Atlas of epilepsies. London: Springer; 2010. p. 1559–62.
5. Shorvon S, Perucca E, Engel J Jr, editors. The treatment of epilepsy. 3rd ed. Oxford: Willey-Blackwell; 2009. p. 1–1056.
6. Shorvon SD. Drug treatment of epilepsy in the century of the ILAE: the second 50 years, 1959-2009. Epilepsia. 2009a;50(Suppl 3):93–130.
7. Shorvon SD. Drug treatment of epilepsy in the century of the ILAE: the first 50 years, 1909-1958. Epilepsia. 2009b;50(Suppl 3):69–92.
8. Wyllie E, Gupta A, Lachhwani D, editors. The treatment of epilepsy. Principles and practice. 4th ed. Philadelphia: Lippincott Williams & Wilkins; 2006.
9. Panayiotopoulos CP. Principles of therapy in the epilepsies. London: Springer; 2010.
10. Patsalos PN, Berry DJ, Bourgeois BF, Cloyd JC, Glauser TA, Johannessen SI, et al. Antiepileptic drugs—best practice guidelines for therapeutic drug monitoring: a position paper by the subcommission on therapeutic drug monitoring, ILAE Commission on Therapeutic Strategies. Epilepsia. 2008;49:1239–76.

# Comorbidities in Epilepsy

**16**

**Abstract**

Comorbidities are additional to epilepsy health and psychosocial problems in a person with epilepsy. Many general medical, neurological and psychosocial disorders occur more frequently in people with epilepsy in comparison to healthy population. Psychiatric (depression, anxiety), cognitive and psychosocial comorbidities prevail. The high rate of comorbidities in epilepsy is mainly attributed to the effects of recurrent seizures, multiple medications, and adverse social reactions to epilepsy such as stigma. Comorbidities in epilepsy often require a multidisciplinary approach to management. Psychological therapies for patients and families are often needed.

**Keywords**

Depression • Anxiety • Cognitive impairment • Stigma • Psychosocial • Prevention • Early identification • Treatment

## What Are Comorbidities in Epilepsy?

Comorbidities are additional to epilepsy health and psychosocial problems in a person with epilepsy.

Scientifically, comorbidity is defined as the combination in a patient of two or more diseases, pathogenetically related to each other or coexisting in a single patient independent of each disease's activity in the patient.

## What Are the Types of Comorbidity in Epilepsy?

Many general medical, neurological and psychosocial disorders occur more frequently in people with epilepsy in comparison to healthy population [1].

**Physical comorbidities,** range from migraine to sleep disorders, cerebrovascular disease, fractures and other injuries, respiratory, cardiac, gastric and intestinal, genital and urinary, dermatological disorders to chronic fatigue. These occur about 20–60% more often in people with epilepsy [2, 3]. Impairment of reproductive function is a very significant but often neglected comorbidity on epilepsy: loss of libido, impotence and infertility can be caused by epilepsy itself, by chronic use of antiepileptic drugs or both [4].

Poor fitness and obesity are also reported at higher rates in epilepsy.

**Neurobehavioural comorbidities** include cognitive impairment, psychiatric disorders, and social problems.

**Cognitive comorbidities** are learning problems that cause difficulty in school and can have lasting effects on educational and professional success.

**Psychiatric comorbidities** are behavior and mood problems which are frequent in patients with epilepsy and have a significant impact on medical management and quality of life. These include depression, anxiety, psychosis, inattention, attention deficit disorder, obsession, personality traits, aggression and suicide alone or more often in combination [5–8]. Psychotic disorders are the less frequent psychiatric comorbidities, but their prevalence rates are still significantly higher than those of the general population. Psychosis of epilepsy can be divided into interictal psychosis of epilepsy, peri-ictal, of which postictal psychosis is the most frequently recognized. Ictal psychotic episodes, present as an expression of non-convulsive status epilepticus. Ictal are the events that happen during a seizure; pre-ictal are the events that happen before a seizure starts; postictal are the events that happen after the end of a seizure.

**Psycho-social comorbidities** are the result of having to deal with the stigma that surrounds epilepsy, the experience of having seizures in public, the difficulty of peer relationships and the discrimination that people with epilepsy often encounter in schools, jobs, sports and social settings (see Chap. 19 on "Metamyth" Psychological Therapy for People who have Epilepsy and 25 on stigma) [9].

## What Are the Causes of Comorbidity in Epilepsy?

The causes of comorbidity in epilepsy are multiple and in general can be divided to:

- "resultant" comorbidities which are the consequence of repeated seizures or treatments
- "causal" that pre-exist and contribute to the development of epilepsy [10].

Comorbidities in epilepsy are traditionally thought to arise predominantly from the effects of recurrent seizures, iatrogenic effects of medications, and adverse social reactions to epilepsy (for example stigma). However, there is a growing body of evidence that other factors are also involved and these include altered neurodevelopment of the brain, cognition, and behaviour; exacerbation of the comorbidities by the chronic effect of medically intractable epilepsy and possible acceleration of common age-associated changes [11]. Lowered seizure threshold may also predispose toward other disorders such as depression, cognitive impairment, sleep disorders, and migraine. Recent research indicates that some cognitive and psychological comorbidities, depression, school problems actually predate the onset of seizures, thus it appears that in some patients epilepsy and certain comorbidities are caused by and reflect the same brain disorder.

Earlier the onset of seizures, severe epilepsy, difficult to control the seizures, and multiple AED medications are significant contributing factors to behavioural and cognition comorbidities.

## The Diagnosis of Comorbidities Is Significant But Often Challenging

Many general medical and neurological conditions occur more frequently in people with epilepsy in comparison to people without epilepsy. Thus, the presence of epilepsy should increase, not reduce, the suspicion that other disorders might be present.

The challenge is to recognize any other disease(s) that might be present in a patient with epilepsy. Fifty percent of people with poorly controlled or other complicated epilepsy have psychiatric or behavioural comorbidities.

For the patient and family, comorbidities are often erroneously considered as the price they have to pay for their epilepsy for the reduction of seizures which is often their main concern.

At the National Institutes of Health conference "Curing Epilepsy 2007: Translating Discoveries into Therapies", the prevention and reversal of the comorbidities of epilepsy were identified as a major new benchmark area for research.

## What Is the Management of Comorbidities in Epilepsy?

Comorbidities often require a multidisciplinary approach to management that is demanding and often frustrating for the family and the treating health care professionals. Their management requires their identification and proper assessment by experts in the field that is affected. It should be realized that an epileptologist is an expert in the diagnosis and management of epilepsy but may not be best qualified for the assessment and treatment of psychological comorbidities that need the support of adequate mental health services. Collaborating with psychiatrists, psychologists and psychotherapists, results in successful assessment and management of epilepsy.

A management strategy should include the following elements:

- Assessment and treatment of epileptic seizures with appropriate medications and probably with non pharmacological methods
- Assessment and treatment of comorbidities by experts in the affected field (mental health professionals for psychiatric disorders)
- treatment of behavioural and cognitive problems with appropriate educational programmers
- family support
- combatting stigma and discrimination.

The difficulty is of how to wholly evaluate the state of a patient who suffers from a number of diseases simultaneously, where to start from and which disease requires primary and subsequent treatment.

*Failures in the management of comorbidities is because parents and patients often do not recognize and report them or what and how to request appropriate help from their health care professionals, because of lack of appropriate information as well as the shortage of specialist services and available resources.*

Because certain comorbidities share an underlying aetiology with epilepsy or can worsen seizure control, treating them will reduce the severity of seizures as well. Conversely, the successful treatment of seizures may reduce the severity of certain comorbidities, such as mood and anxiety disorders [1].

Children that live in a well organised and well disciplined family are better able to compensate for some of the cognitive deficits, do better than anticipated in school and do not have as many behavioural or mental health problems.

Depression, learning and behavioural abnormalities may occur in patients with epilepsy in remission. These may be patients who did not get the appropriate social, medical, educational and psychological attention and treatment when they were younger. Thus, early identification of possible risk factors for educational, language, and behavioral problems, and interventions is probably mandatory in addition to the treatment of epileptic seizures.

## Recommendations to Patients with Epilepsy and Their Family

The majority of people with epilepsy do not have significant comorbidities and they should lead a normal life. However, because comorbidities are sometimes affecting seriously many aspects of health, family, social and work life, it is important that these are identified and reported to health professionals and educators for their treatment. Please, record and put in writing:

- any problems that may pre-existed the onset of epilepsy
- any problems and their progression that appeared with the onset of epilepsy
- any problems and their progression that appeared with the start of antiepileptic drug medication

Convey these and discuss them with your physician, other health professionals, social and educational services. Make sure that these are well understood and not undermined. Check yourself the list of side effects of the used antiepileptic drug to see whether the symptom you are concerned with is listed (some of antiepileptic drug side effects may be rare for most of the patients and therefore not well appreciated by the physicians).

**Remember:**
- Comorbidity of epilepsy refers to the coexistence or co-occurrence of other additional medical, physical, psychological and social problems in a person with epilepsy. These problems can be related or unrelated to the underlying cause of epilepsy, the effect of epileptic seizures and its treatments.
- The identification of co-morbid disorders in a patient with epilepsy is very significant because they pose a significant burden on patients and their quality of life.
- Prevention, early identification, and treatment of comorbid conditions may reduce morbidity, mortality and improve health outcomes in people with epilepsy. Yet comorbidities whether the result of epilepsy or independent of it often remain unrecognized, undiagnosed and untreated because epilepsy prevails in the mind of the treating physicians and the patient is reluctant or does not speak about them.
- Management strategies employed in the outpatient clinic to maximize overall health outcomes should include screening and treatment for the commonly coexistent conditions in persons with epilepsy.
- Patients and family should be aware and report comorbidities to their health care professionals because these need medical or psychological attention for treatment.

## Recommended Readings

- Epilepsy Foundation. Comorbidities in Epilepsy: http://www.epilepsyfoundation.org/aboutepilepsy/relatedconditions/Comorbidites-in-Epilepsy.cfm
- http://www.epilepsy.com/information/professionals/co-existing-disorders
- http://www.epilepsy.com/information/professionals/joint-content-partnership-aes/epilepsy-comorbidities
- Epilepsy and neuropsychiatric comorbidities http://apt.rcpsych.org/content/17/1/44

## References

1. Wiebe S, Hesdorffer DC. Epilepsy: being ill in more ways than one. Epilepsy Curr. 2007;7:145–8.
2. Gaitatzis A, Carroll K, Majeed A, Sander W. The epidemiology of the comorbidity of epilepsy in the general population. Epilepsia. 2004;45:1613–22.

3. Gaitatzis A. The comorbidity of epilepsy: epidemiology, mechanisms and consequences. In: Panayiotopoulos CP, editor. Atlas of epilepsies. London: Springer; 2010. p. 1325–9.
4. Verrotti A, Loiacono G, Laus M, Coppola G, Chiarelli F, Tiboni GM. Hormonal and reproductive disturbances in epileptic male patients: emerging issues. Reprod Toxicol. 2011;31:519–27.
5. Hamed SA. Psychiatric symptomatologies and disorders related to epilepsy and antiepileptic medications. Expert Opin Drug Saf. 2011;10:913–34.
6. Kanner AM. Common psychiatric comorbidities in epilepsy: epidemiologic, pathogenic and clinical aspects. In: Panayiotopoulos CP, editor. Atlas of epilepsies. London: Springer; 2010. p. 1337–44.
7. Kanner AM. Treatment of comorbid psychiatric disorders in epilepsy: a review of practical strategies. In: Panayiotopoulos CP, editor. Atlas of epilepsies. London: Springer; 2010.
8. Kimiskidis VK, Valeta T. Epilepsy and anxiety: epidemiology, classification, aetiology, and treatment. Epileptic Disord. 2012;14:248–56.
9. Valeta T, de Boer HM. Stigma and discrimination in epilepsy. In: Panayiotopoulos CP, editor. Atlas of epilepsies. London: Springer; 2010. p. 1363–6.
10. Duchowny MS, Bourgeois B. Coexisting disorders in children with epilepsy. Adv Stud Med. 2003;3(7B):S680–S83.
11. Hermann B, Seidenberg M, Jones J. The neurobehavioural comorbidities of epilepsy: can a natural history be developed? Lancet Neurol. 2008;7:151–60.

# Psychogenic Non-Epileptic Seizures

# 17

**Abstract**

Psychogenic non-epileptic seizures are non-epileptic attacks resembling an epileptic seizure, but without the characteristic electrical discharges associated with epilepsy. They are stress-related or emotional and result from traumatic psychological experiences. Psychogenic non-epileptic seizures are mainly convulsive and occur in wakefulness and in the presence of witnesses. They are commonly confused and misdiagnosed as genuine epileptic seizures. Outcome is generally good if diagnosis is made early and psychological treatment is taken.

**Keywords**

Pseudo-seizures • Hysteric attacks • Stress-related • Psychological trauma • Panic • Psychotherapy • Anxiety • Depression • Inductions • Video-EEG

## What Are Psychogenic Seizures?

Psychogenic seizures or preferably psychogenic non-epileptic seizures (PNES) are non-epileptic attacks resembling an epileptic seizure, but without the characteristic electrical discharges associated with epilepsy [1–4]. They look-like but they are not genuine epileptic seizures. They are stress-related or emotional and result from traumatic psychological experiences [5]. They are sometimes called pseudoseizures (or hysterical attacks). This term is discouraged because PNES are not 'pseudo' that is they are not faked. Freud in 1924 writing about Dostoevsky's epilepsy says that it is right to distinguish between an "organic" and an "affective epilepsy". "In the first case the mental life of the patient is subjected to an alien disturbance from without in the second case the disturbance is an expression of his mental life itself" [6].

© Springer International Publishing AG 2017
T. Valeta, *The Epilepsy Book: A Companion for Patients*,
DOI 10.1007/978-3-319-61679-7_17

PNES are extremely real episodes they are not voluntary and can be very troublesome to a person's life and have their own stigma. Their distinction from epileptic seizures is based on clinical history and manifestations and more definitely when recorded with video-EEG.

## What Are the Clinical Manifestations of Psychogenic Seizures?

Individuals experiencing PNES may display a variety of symptoms which may be:

(a) convulsive
(b) non-convulsive
(c) panic

The duration of PNES is usually longer than the epileptic seizures. They usually last over 10 min to some hours.

**Convulsive PNES** manifest with convulsions like the generalised tonic clonic epileptic seizures [1]. These involve dropping to the floor with movements of arms, legs, head and trunk. Movements are usually asymmetrical and asynchronous, accelerating and decelerating, stop and go, bicycling, arching of the back, forward pelvic thrusting, side-to-side shaking of the head, tightly closed eyelids with resistance to attempts to passive opening. There may be weeping, stuttering and vocalizations. The patient appears but is not unconscious. Most patients show signs of being able to react to their environment and some may be able to talk whilst having an attack and follow commands.

A few patients may flip on one side and fall on the ground, remain still and unresponsive, thus mimicking syncope rather than epilepsy.

## What Are the Main Differences in the Manifestations of Convulsive PNES from Genuine Generalized Convulsive Epileptic Seizures?

Psychogenic seizures:

- Are often precipitated by stressful circumstances though stress is also a precipitating factor in epilepsy
- Can be induced in response to suggestion (useful in diagnostic provocative activating techniques also called 'inductions')
- Occur in wakefulness and often in the presence of witnesses
- 'Convulsions' may be interrupted or resistant to restraint
- Eyes are commonly closed (probably the most important symptom to enable differentiation from GTCSs and syncopes, where the eyes are invariably open)
- Attempts to open the eyes passively often result in tightening of the eyelids
- Distress and behaviours exhibited during the attacks
- The patient may become emotional and cry after the end of the non-epileptic seizure
- Post-ictal behaviour of responding to questions in a whispered voice or responding to commands with semi-motor responses

**In the non-convulsive PNES** people go blank with temporary loss of attention or stare. They may not move at all, or only move a little. These attacks resemble epileptic complex focal or absence seizures.

Difficulty in breathing, palpitations and increased perspiration are common in any type of PNES.

**Panic Attacks** are of abrupt onset, manifesting with an intense sense of extreme fear often with trembling, shortness of breath, heart palpitations, chest pain, sweating, dizziness, hyperventilation, numbness, nausea or vomiting, or sensations of choking. Panic attacks are actually a fight-or-flight response occurring out of context or as a response to minimal provocative factors. Patients suffer from panic, other anxiety disorders or phobias. Psychogenic non-epileptic panic attacks should mainly be differentiated from simple focal seizures of mesial temporal lobe epilepsy.

## What Are Common Triggers of Psychogenic Seizures?

Emotional triggers such as stress, argumentative conversations, conflicts and becoming upset are common in PNES.

## What Is the Aetiology of Psychogenic Seizures?

Psychogenic seizures are epileptic-like physical manifestations of a psychological disturbance. They are currently classified as a conversion disorder, according to the Diagnostic and Statistical Manual of Mental Disorders, fifth edition (DSM-5). Conversion is a somatoform disorder (taking form in the body) manifesting with physical symptoms caused by psychological conflict, unconsciously converted to resemble those of a neurologic disorder. In other words, PNES are caused by an unconscious conversion of emotional distress into physical symptoms. Patients with PNES have high rates of repressed anger, traumatic sexual experience and life stressors often blocked from consciousness; patients can recall the underlying events only with help from a trained therapist. The unconscious processes that cause PNES may also cause or contribute to other conditions, such as depression, anxiety, emotional stress, rage, fear and panic, in addition to other mental disturbances.

Patients with psychogenic seizures are not faking illness; they sincerely believe that they have a serious physical problem. A seizure is a way to express what the mouth and mind cannot express.

## How Common Are Psychogenic Seizures and at What Age They Occur? Epidemiology

Patients with PNES make up approximately 20% of those referred to specialist epilepsy clinics.

They usually start in young adulthood and occur more frequently in women than in men at a ratio 4 to 1.

## How Psychogenic Seizures Are Diagnosed? Evaluation and Tests

Psychogenic seizures are diagnosed on clinical evidence by its triggers and presentation. They are confirmed by obtaining video EEG recordings of the events.

## What Is the Management of Psychogenic Seizures?

Psychogenic seizures need urgent and skillful treatment, which is often successful, particularly if they are recognised and managed during the early stages. The role of the health carer is not just simply to announce to the patient: 'You do not suffer from epileptic seizures'. At this stage, the patient requires a thorough and tactful explanation of what this new diagnosis of PNES means and the appropriate management procedures. These patients have been allowed to believe for many years that they suffered from 'epilepsy' that was intractable to medication. Their reaction and that of their family to a new diagnosis of 'psychogenic seizures' (also taking into consideration the negative social implications and attitudes to this term) should be thoroughly considered. It is also important to present a PNES diagnosis with care because some patients would react with aggressive denial or suicidal behavior. A patient who believes that he or she has been perceived as a liar or "fake" may feel humiliated. In a substantial number of patients (around 50%) a proper explanation of the diagnosis, particularly with the help of the video-recorded events, stops the attacks [7]. However, long-term outcome studies in PNES show that a significant proportion of patients remains symptomatic and experiences continued impairments in quality of life and functionality.

It is important that people suffering with PNES should know that there is hope and that people with PNES can be treated with psychotherapy. Neurology, psychiatry and psychology should work together with the patient, so we can contribute into finding treatments to relieve those patients from suffering [8].

People with comorbid issues such as anxiety and depression may be given medication and undertake psychotherapy. Effective coping strategies for these conditions can be offered.

## What Is the Long Term Outcome (Prognosis) and Evolution of PNES?

Overall, the outcome is good. With proper treatment, up to 40% of treated PNES patients remain event-free for a median of 5 years, the attacks eventually disappear in 60–70% of adults.

Favourable prognostic factors include being female, effective early intervention, normal premorbid psychological make-up, and good family support.

An important factor is early diagnosis and management. The shorter patients have carried the wrong diagnosis of epilepsy, the better the chances of full recovery.

The outcome of PNES is generally better in children and adolescents than in adults, probably because the duration of illness is shorter and the psychopathology or stressors are different in paediatric patients than in adults.

## Recommendations for Patients and Family

The main recommendation is to make sure that you have the right diagnosis. Do you truly have PNES or is this epilepsy or something else? If you have PNES find out what may be the cause of it and get the best possible management by experienced and well qualified psychiatrist/psychotherapist.

## Recommended Readings

- Non-Epileptic attacks. This site provides patients diagnosed with PNES and their families useful information about the disorder. http://www.nonepilepticattacks.info/
- Benbadis SR, Heriaud L, Psychogenic (Non-Epileptic)Seizures, A Guide for Families & Patients. http://hsc.usf.edu/COM/epilepsy/PNESbrochure.pdf
  See also other websites at:
- https://www.ncbi.nlm.nih.gov/pmc/articles/PMC3523560/
- https://www.epilepsysociety.org.uk/non-epileptic-seizures#.WKMnt_l97IU
- http://www.goodtherapy.org/blog/psychpedia/psychogenic-nonepileptic-seizures
- https://www.ncbi.nlm.nih.gov/pmc/articles/PMC3931180/
- http://www.sciencedirect.com/science/article/pii/S1525505010006694
- http://ac.els-cdn.com/S030384670800334X/1-s2.0-S030384670800334X-main.pdf?_tid=78537878-f2d1-11e6-8c74-00000aab0f6c&acdnat=1487089396_927532a8a7f012786ab969b95f23279a

## References

1. Reuber M, Brown RJ. Understanding psychogenic nonepileptic seizures-phenomenology, semiology and the integrative cognitive model. Seizure. 2017;44:199–205.
2. Doss RC, LaFrance WC Jr. Psychogenic non-epileptic seizures. Epileptic Disord. 2016;18:337–43.
3. Lesser RP. Psychogenic seizures. Neurology. 1996;46:1499–507.
4. Brown RJ, Syed TU, Benbadis S, LaFrance WC Jr, Reuber M. Psychogenic nonepileptic seizures. Epilepsy Behav. 2011;22:85–93.
5. Valeta T. The potential of dramatherapy in the treatment of epilepsy. MA Thesis, University of Derby; 2009.
6. Freud S (orig.1928) An autobiographical study, inhibitions, symptoms and anxiety, lay analysis, and other works, vol. 5. London: Vintage; 2001.
7. Wiseman H, Mousa S, Howlett S, Reuber M. A multicenter evaluation of a brief manualized psychoeducation intervention for psychogenic nonepileptic seizures delivered by health professionals with limited experience in psychological treatment. Epilepsy Behav. 2016;63:50–6.

8. Valeta T. 'Metamyth' © and Dramatherapy: an innovative approach for people with epilepsy. In: Schrader C, editor. Ritual theatre. The power of dramatic ritual in personal development groups and clinical practice. London: Jessica Kingsley; 2012. p. 275–90.

# Psychological Treatments for Epilepsy

**18**

### Abstract

Various types of psychological treatments (psychotherapy) have been applied in epilepsy with the aim of alleviating psychiatric comorbidities, reducing seizures or both. Seizure-precipitants can be modified appropriately to reduce seizures. The type of psychotherapy used will depend on your personal needs and which method your psychotherapist thinks will be most helpful for resolving your issues. Although all types of psychotherapy can be effective, you may find one approach more appealing than another, or find that some approaches are better for a certain area of counselling or psychotherapy than others. Psychobehavioural therapies are most extensively applied in epilepsy. They include cognitive behavioural therapy, behavioural and mind-body approaches Cognitive behavioural play therapy. The Arts therapies (music therapy, dramatherapy, movement therapy and art therapy) are psychotherapies using the arts as a medium for expression of feelings that are not accessible by other means. Metamyth©/Dramatherapy is an innovative approach to Dramatherapy which is used as a psychological treatment for people who have epilepsy as well as for any psychiatric disorders.

### Keywords

Psychotherapy • Psychobehavioural therapies • Cognitive behavioural therapy • Psychodynamic psychoanalytic psychotherapy • Psychoanalytic psychotherapy • Mind-body therapy • Arts therapies • Music therapy • Metamyth©/Dramatherapy

## Why People with Epilepsy Need Psychological Treatments?

Many people with epilepsy struggle with feelings of anxiety, depression, low self-esteem, difficulties in relations, employment and stigma. Various types of psychological treatments (psychotherapy) have been applied in epilepsy with the aim of improving the quality of life of patients by alleviating psychiatric comorbidities, reducing seizures or both. The rationale for this is that (a) psychiatric comorbidities and particularly depression and anxiety have a detrimental effect in the quality of life as well as increasing the risk for seizures and (b) seizure-precipitants can be modified appropriately to reduce seizures.

Together with medication, psychotherapy is aiming to improve the quality of life for patients with epilepsy.

## What Is Psychotherapy?

Psychotherapy is the use of psychological methods, to help a person change and overcome problems, improve an individual's wellbeing and resolve or mitigate troublesome behaviours, beliefs, compulsions, thoughts, or emotions, and to improve relationships and social skills.

Some therapists teach specific skills to help you tolerate painful emotions, manage relationships more effectively, or improve behaviour. You may also be encouraged to develop your own solutions.

There is individual or group psychotherapy.

## What Are the Various Types of Psychotherapy?

There are many different types of psychotherapy. The type used will depend on your personal needs and which method your psychotherapist thinks will be most helpful for resolving your issues. Although all types of psychotherapy can be effective, you may find one approach more appealing than another, or find that some approaches are better for a certain area of counselling or psychotherapy than others. Psychotherapy encourages you to explore your physical symptoms and your emotions by relating them to both current and past experiences in your life. Through this you may become able to recognise and process the impact of difficult events and situations, improving your ability to deal with the challenges of daily life. You may be referred to a named psychotherapist by your doctor, but if you have to look for one yourself, make sure that you select a member of a formal professional association.

Some of the main types of psychotherapy in epilepsy are outlined below. Alternative remedies for epilepsy such as spirituality, energy healing, aromatherapy, although they appear to be psychological in nature, will not be included here.

## Psychobehavioural Therapies

Psychobehavioural therapies are most extensively applied in epilepsy. They include cognitive behavioural therapy, behavioral and mind-body approaches [1].

## Cognitive Behavioural Therapy (CBT)

This treatment is based on a combination of cognitive and behavioural psychotherapy [2, 3].

Cognitive therapy explores ways your thoughts and beliefs may be causing emotional problems. Your therapist will discuss these issues with you so you can try to develop more helpful ways of thinking to allow you to overcome your problems.

Behavioural psychotherapy involves finding ways to help you change the way you act. It is often used to overcome a specific fear by encouraging you to gradually face these fears and help you relax and feel comfortable as you do it. In epilepsy, it operates by applying countermeasures upon seizure triggers and aura interruption at the early stages of seizure activity to abort or reduce the likelihood of developing a seizure from the outset.

Cognitive–behavioural interventions targets cognitive structures and distortions that maintain symptoms of anxiety and depression. Correction of those dysfunctional concepts leads to clinical improvement and prevention of recurrence. During CBT, you and your therapist agree on tasks for you to do in between sessions. This will help you deal with problems yourself, so you no longer need therapy.

## Cognitive Behavioural Play Therapy

Cognitive behavioural play therapy is commonly used with children. By watching children play, therapists are able to gain insight into what a child is uncomfortable expressing or unable to express. Children may be able to choose their own toys and play freely. They might be asked to draw a picture or use toys to create scenes in a sandbox. Therapists may teach parents how to use play to improve communication with their children.

## Psychodynamic (Psychoanalytic) Psychotherapy

Psychodynamic therapy is a less intensive form of psychoanalysis that uses similar techniques, but aims to find quicker solutions to more immediate problems. Art, music, drama and movement therapies often use the psychodynamic model of working, but encourage alternative forms of self-expression and communication as well as talking. Musical or technical skills or experience in drama and movement are not needed for this type of therapy to be successful.

## Cognitive Analytical Therapy

During early sessions of cognitive analytical therapy, you'll discuss events and experiences from your past to help you understand why you feel, think and behave the way you do now.

After the first few sessions, your therapist will write down what you have discussed on paper, and will work with you to map out problem patterns that have emerged to help you understand how these problems occurred. Your therapist will use this to help you figure out ways of changing these problem patterns. They may suggest using diaries and progress charts to help you develop skills you can use to continue improving after the therapy sessions have finished.

## Mind-Body Approaches

Mindfulness and acceptance-based meditation are common mind-body approaches used in patients with epilepsy [4]. Mindfulness meditation is a practice that aims at focusing one's awareness on the present moment. They involve self-observation of mental and bodily activity, attention training and the cultivation of process-oriented awareness. The therapeutic components of mindfulness are to acquire attention control by focusing on internal processes and external stimuli at the present moment ("here-and-now"), with non-elaborative attitude and non-judgemental acceptance. These techniques have been formalized into standardized psychotherapy such as Mindfulness Based Stress Reduction, Mindfulness Based Cognitive Therapy and Acceptance and Commitment Therapy.

## Arts Psychotherapies

The Arts therapies (music therapy, art therapy, dramatherapy and movement therapy) are psychotherapies using the arts as a medium for expression of feelings that are not accessible by other means. The nature of the arts experience and relationships within the arts therapies is seen to offer specific opportunities to the client. The arts therapies can be seen, as a way to reflect, encounter and transform unconscious material that is part of a problematic situation for the client.

The main tradition that the arts therapies have drawn on has been one that separates each art form through training, methods and processes that are distinct. These are seen to be specific to the art form and are separate from one another. However there are examples of arts therapists within this tradition using aspects of the arts outside their own "domain". This tends to involve using a part of the language of another art and drawing it into their own art form. Importantly, though, the process has not just to do with the creation of opportunities for access. The process of expression and the process of creativity along with contact with others, or the therapist, are seen as crucial to the process of change.

Dramatherapy is the use of drama and theatre processes to achieve therapeutic goals. Dramatherapy is used in a variety of settings including hospitals, schools, mental health centres, prisons and businesses thus treating individuals with a range of mental health, cognitive and developmental disorders. Metamyth©/Dramatherapy is an innovative approach to dramatherapy which is used as a psychological treatment for people who have epilepsy as well as any psychiatric disorder (see Chap. 19) [5, 6].

Music Therapy is consisting of a process in which a music therapist uses music in all its facets physical, emotional, mental, social, aesthetic, and spiritual to help clients improve their physical and mental health (music therapy-Wikipedia at https://en.wikipedia.org/wiki/Music_therapy).

Art Therapy uses the creative process of making art, to improve a person's physical, mental, and emotional wellbeing. The creative process with the presence of the therapist may assist individuals as they address areas of difficulty or concern.

Dance Movement Psychotherapy is a relational process in which a client and therapist engage in an empathetic, creative process, using body movement and dance, to assist the integration of emotional, cognitive, physical, social and spiritual aspects of self.

## Other Types of Psychotherapy

**Interpersonal psychotherapy** focuses on the individual and his/her primary social group in relationship to one another and their circumstances or environment. Their beliefs, attitudes, and expectations about what is "normal," as well as associated emotions and meanings, are addressed in counseling to help them reach optimum person-in relationship- in environment congruence. This psychotherapy is recommended for depression.

**Integrated somatoform psychotherapies** (e.g., Eye Movement Desensitization and Reprocessing, EMDR) are client paced and focus on affective, cognitive, and somatic perceptual components of trauma in its various forms and anxiety disorders. The processing tools include both desensitization to stimuli that trigger present distress as a result of second order conditioning and change in cognitions from negative (succumbing) to positive (thriving).

## Humanistic Therapies

Humanistic therapies encourage you to explore how you think about yourself and recognise your strengths. The aim is to help you think about yourself more positively and improve your self-awareness.

There are a several types of humanistic therapies, which are described below.

- **person-centred counselling**—aims to create a non-judgmental environment where you can feel comfortable talking about yourself and are able to see that you have the ability to change. Your therapist will try to look at your experiences from your point of view.

- **Gestalt therapy**—takes a holistic approach, focusing on your experiences, thoughts, feelings and actions to help improve your self-awareness.
- **transactional analysis**—aims to explore how the problems in your life may have been shaped by decisions and teachings from childhood. You'll work with your therapist to help you find ways to break away from these unconscious repetitive patterns of thinking and behaving.
- **transpersonal psychology**—encourages you to explore who you really are as a person. It often involves using techniques such as meditation and visualisation.
- **existential therapy**—aims to help increase your self-awareness and make sense of your existence. Existential therapy is not too concerned with your past, but instead focuses on the choices to be made in the present and future.

## Family and Couple (Systemic) Therapy

Family therapy focuses on family relationships, such as marriage, and encourages everyone within the family or relationship to work together to fix problems.

The therapist encourages group discussions or exercises that involve everyone, and promotes a healthy family unit as a way of improving mental health.

## Supportive Counseling

Supportive counseling is an essential element in each of the above psychotherapies and leads to better coping. Its key components include a conversational style, creating a therapeutic alliance, enhancing the patient's self-esteem through praise or appropriate reassurance, reducing anxiety by providing anticipatory guidance and advice, and enhancing adaptive skills through clarification and gentle confrontation.

## Is Psychotherapy Beneficial for People with Epilepsy?

The prevailing view is that psychotherapy is beneficial for people with epilepsy if appropriately tailored to the needs of the patient (see Chap. 19 on "Metamyth"©) and skillfully performed by well-trained therapists [7, 8]. Psychotherapy is particularly useful for patients with comorbid depression and anxiety as well as those who also suffer from psychogenic non-epileptic attacks. Seizures can also be reduced by means of eliminating certain epileptic triggers [9].

## Psychosocial and/or Educational Treatment Programs in Epilepsy

Though not psychotherapy, psychosocial and/or educational treatment programs in epilepsy have developed in order to educate patients about the various medico-behaviour and other aspects of epilepsy and encourage them to cope actively with their disease, to live with as few limitations as possible, to participate in the treatment process, and to gain more self-esteem. In my research study investigating parental reactions and needs of children who have Idiopathic focal epilepsies, the parents when asked if they need help other than medical, express the need for education on epilepsy for themselves and their children by 66.7% [10]. (see Chap. 24 on Parental Reactions and Needs in Idiopathic Focal Epilepsies).

The educational treatment programs have resulted in a reduction of psychosocial problems and an improvement of quality of life in patients with epilepsy [11]. Thus, epilepsy education helps people with epilepsy become self-confident, competent in self-management, aware of their needs, and able to access resources to meet their needs—thus it helps them become better partners in patient-centered care. Moreover, having accurate, in-depth information about epilepsy helps people better understand the disorder, prevents misconceptions, and reduces concerns about stigma. Finally, epilepsy education helps promote optimal well-being and quality of life.

Educating patients and their families through seminars, courses and lectures is essential in order to reduce anxiety, panic and psychosocial morbidity in those affected. Child-centered, family-focused counselling models for parents are used to help them deal with their anger, resentment, grief and anxiety, and thus contribute to effective child care [12].

## Recommended Readings

- The epilepsy psychotherapy service http://www.sth.nhs.uk/clientfiles/File/pd5335_EpilepsyPsychologyService.pdf
- Psychological treatments for people with epilepsy http://onlinelibrary.wiley.com/doi/10.1002/14651858.CD012081/full
- Psychotherapies http://www.rcpsych.ac.uk/healthadvice/treatmentswellbeing/psychotherapies.aspx
- Educating People with Epilepsy and Their Families https://www.ncbi.nlm.nih.gov/books/NBK100608/
- Educational programs in epilepsy http://www.epilepsy.com/get-help/services-and-support/education-programs
- British Association of Dramatherapy http://www.badth.org.uk
- Art Therapy http://www.arttherapyblog.com
- Dance Movement Psychotherapy http://www.roehampton.ac.uk/dance/

# References

1. Tang V, Michaelis R, Kwan P. Psychobehavioral therapy for epilepsy. Epilepsy Behav. 2014;32:147–55.
2. Carbone L, Plegue M, Barnes A, Shellhaas R. Improving the mental health of adolescents with epilepsy through a group cognitive behavioral therapy program. Epilepsy Behav. 2014;39:130–4.
3. Gandy M, Karin E, Fogliati VJ, McDonald S, Titov N, Dear BF. A feasibility trial of an Internet-delivered and transdiagnostic cognitive behavioral therapy treatment program for anxiety, depression, and disability among adults with epilepsy. Epilepsia. 2016;57:1887–96.
4. Tang V, Poon WS, Kwan P. Mindfulness-based therapy for drug-resistant epilepsy: an assessor-blinded randomized trial. Neurology. 2015;85:1100–7.
5. Valeta T. The potential of dramatherapy in the treatment of epilepsy. MA thesis, University of Derby; 2009.
6. Valeta T. 'Metamyth'© and Dramatherapy: an innovative approach for people with epilepsy. In: Schrader C, editor. Ritual theatre. The power of dramatic ritual in personal development groups and clinical practice. London: Jessica Kingsley; 2012. p. 275–90.
7. Goldstein LH, McAlpine M, Deale A, Toone BK, Mellers JD. Cognitive behaviour therapy with adults with intractable epilepsy and psychiatric co-morbidity: preliminary observations on changes in psychological state and seizure frequency. Behav Res Ther. 2003;41:447–60.
8. Kelley SDM. Psychological therapies in epilepsy. In: Panayiotopoulos CP, editor. Atlas of epilepsies. London: Springer; 2010. p. 1693–5.
9. Wolf P. From precipitation to inhibition of seizures: rationale of a therapeutic paradigm. Epilepsia. 2005;46(Suppl 1):15–6.
10. Valeta T. Psychological aspects, parental reactions and needs in idiopathic focal epilepsies. Epileptic Disord. 2016;18:19–22.
11. Mittan RJ. Psychosocial treatment programs in epilepsy: a review. Epilepsy Behav. 2009;16:371–80.
12. Valeta T, Sogawa Y, Moshe SL. Impact of focal seizures on patients and family. In: Panayiotopoulos CP, Benbadis S, Sisodiya S, editors. Focal epilepsies: seizures, syndromes and management, vol. 5. Oxford: Medicinae; 2008. p. 230–8.

# "Metamyth"©/Dramatherapy

**19**

**Abstract**

"Metamyth"©/Dramatherapy is a psychological therapy for people who have epilepsy. "Metamyth"© can be used for any client population at any age or stage of development. "Metamyth"© is unique, as it is a psychological treatment conceived by taking into consideration, the clinical experience and knowledge from researching epilepsy and by exploring the archetypal dimensions of the psyche of the person who has epilepsy, studying the psychological needs of this group, and adapting psychotherapeutic processes.

**Keywords**

Metamyth©Dramatherapy • Psychotherapy • Epilepsy • Psychiatric disorders • Patients

## What Is Metamyth©?

"Metamyth"© is a psychological treatment for people who have epilepsy. Metamyth© is an action psychotherapy, that has drawn upon arts based approaches and Dramatherapy, Psychodrama, a Mind and Body approach and a Neurobiological approach to Psychology and Therapy. It is influenced by humanistic Jungian and existential psychotherapies and it is psychoanalytically oriented [1].

"Metamyth"© is both therapy and art and has a poetic basis to contribute to the thinking and practice of therapy. It makes use of all the arts and draws from the historic use of the connection of the arts and healing.

Working with people who have epilepsy and medical specialists, it became clear to me that they were very serious limits in the approach of the medical model and that epilepsy can have a profound emotional impact on the whole family

© Springer International Publishing AG 2017
T. Valeta, *The Epilepsy Book: A Companion for Patients*,
DOI 10.1007/978-3-319-61679-7_19

surrounding the person or those affected. I worked very hard independently to pursue my interest in the missing pieces of the jigsaw puzzle [1].

My research confirmed my observation and I moved into the third stage of my involvement, that of how I can help specifically, to meet the needs of people who have epilepsy.

I have attempted to bring together with the medical model the psychological approach "Metamyth"© as a treatment to help alleviate the symptoms of epilepsy by (a) reducing the frequency of seizures and (b) by improving the overall health and well being of the individual and their family.

The creation of "Metamyth"© is an investigation into the relationship between depth psychology (psychologies that take unconscious process into account) epilepsy and Dramatherapy [1].

This approach is informed by the field of neurology and psychotherapy, as well as my meetings and exchanges with neurologists, psychiatrists, psychotherapists, psychoanalysts and Arts Therapists who have supported me and influenced this work. Working with individuals who have epilepsy has been an inspiration to this model which I currently offer as complimentary to medical treatment.

## Etymology and Meaning of the Word "Metamyth"©

I invented the word "Metamyth"© [2] from the Greek language, and its meaning is the center of the work. Etymologically the prefix meta means, after, in modern Greek and, with, in ancient Greek. Together with the word myth it means, with the myth and after the myth. I made up the word "Metamyth"© because *I see that from the moment a person enters therapy the togetherness of the therapist with the client creates a myth of its own. The meaning of the word "Metamyth"© expresses the companionship and togetherness of the patient and therapist to create a relationship of trust and openness, a myth, which then, meta, will lead to another way of being of the patient and the therapist. It also means the story, the myth of every person's life during the time it is lived and after the events for which he/she is concerned.* Therefore" Metamyth"© has to do with time with how things have been before during and after. This is a pathos/mythos connection; pathos meaning in Greek, things that have happened, it also means suffering (a difficulty) and mythos is the word for myth. With the word "Metamyth"©, and the meaning it represents, as the center of my work, I help people with epilepsy discover their own potential and resources to heal themselves and make responsible choices based on their abilities and not on their diagnosis as having epilepsy [1].

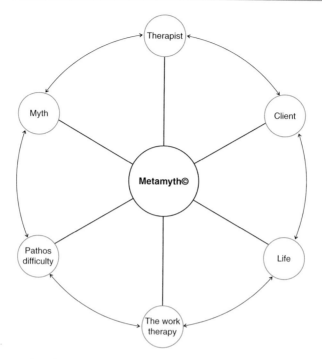

Graphic representation of "Metamyth"© as described in the text above

## "Metamyth"© and Dramatherapy

"Metamyth"© in its philosophy and practice brings together a theatre based approach (Dramatherapy) [3] and a psychodynamic oriented one (Psychoanalysis). The therapeutic aspect of drama, was first acknowledged in the Greek theatre, where philosophy and politics poetry and plays were presented to people of every walk of life. Drama means action in Greek and it is understood in every language as interaction representation, happenings, communication. Theatre is an art. Coming from the word *theoro* which means viewing in Greek it involves actors, stage, audience, performance, interaction, and environment. Metaphorically speaking, a "Metamyth"© session becomes a stage where we explore personal myths and the inner images of the self [1]. This is a creative process. By using metaphor, possibilities are being tried out safely and freely by the individual and awareness and change may happen in an experiential way.

## A "Metamyth"© Session

A"Metamyth"© session has a structure: warm up, focus, main activity, closure deroling, completion. The therapist may have an aim and rationale for why they are using the particular exercises or activities always taking into consideration the needs of the patient's age, vital capacity, stage of life cognitive and psysiological differences, mental health issues, cultural or religious factors, as well as other issues which may be relevant to each individual. Every session is a part of a whole but it also stands on its own as a blue print for the client and therapist as they perform their roles.

A "Metamyth"© therapist needs to be culturally literate in order to contextualize the work within the client's principles, social values, tradition, and the ethos of the setting in which therapy will take place.

"Metamyth"© enables each individual who has epilepsy to self-regulate, psychologically and improve their ability of self-reliance, self-respect, and self-empowerment. The emotional literacy of the individual, is supported by the work,(therapy) which is informed by contemporary affective neuroscience.

## Why Is "Metamyth"© a Unique Psychological Treatment for People with Epilepsy?

"Metamyth"© is unique as it is a psychological treatment conceived by taking into consideration, the clinical experience and knowledge from researching epilepsy and by exploring the archetypal dimensions of the psyche of the person who has epilepsy, studying the psychological needs of this group, and adapting psychotherapeutic processes.

There can be very specific psychological needs at different stages of human development with reference to epilepsy. "Metamyth"© addresses these aspects to facilitate difficulties arising in different age groups.

Psychiatric disorders can be identified in 25–50% of patients with epilepsy, with higher prevalence among patients with poorly controlled seizures. These include depression 11–60%, anxiety 19–45%, psychotic disorders 2–8%, ADHD 25–30% [2]. "Metamyth"© considers diagnosis,recognition and treatment of these disorders in epilepsy patients as essential, in order to improve their quality of life and make the most of their abilities. The medical perspective must be examined in full and in detail before a therapeutic approach could be applied.

A Metamyth© Therapist should be aware of the many types of epileptic seizures including minor seizures (as absences, mild myoclonic jerks, subjective internal sensations as auras, dreamy states, psychic or mental symptoms) which are likely to be unnoticed, in order to recognize them and treat the client with sensitivity during and after this experience.

A Metamyth© therapist should be educated in psychogenic seizures, and trained in what to do if a seizure occurs during therapy. Psychogenic non epileptic seizures [4] result from a variety of psychological disturbances (see Chap. 17). A psychological cause makes the patients believe that they have a physical problem. This is in keeping with most theories of psychoanalysis which suggest neurosis to be the consequence of denied, repressed or neglected aspects of the self [5].

They are difficult to distinguish from epileptic events.

Since the 1930s the psychological aspects of epilepsy have been viewed as important as its physical aspect. Nowadays psychotherapeutic interventions are also regarded as important. I suggest that 'Metamyth'© is especially relevant for the psychogenic type.

People with epilepsy experience a social identity that is vulnerable and at risk from being demolished by a seizure that could burst through at any time. Their self-regulation is compromised by their physical condition and requires additional psychological help.

My objective is to treat the psychological side of the problem and the social implications in order to achieve a better quality of life and in that way potentially reduce the frequency of seizures [1].

Epilepsy has always been associated with social stigma (see chapter on stigma) mainly because of its dramatic manifestation with the seizures where the person falls down jerks or loses conscience. The people diagnosed with epilepsy and their families, feel fear and shame and develop a special 'epileptic identity' [6]. underpinned by these feelings. This leads to isolation and anxiety over negative reactions from other people. Patients are found with greater perceived helpnessness rates of anxiety and depression, somatic symtomatology, and reduced life satisfaction [7]. Some conceal their condition from employers friends or partners for fear of shame, and discrimination. Isolation is also a result of this fear and shame, low self-esteem and self-image. "Metamyth"© will help people who have epilepsy to overcome social stigma and continue their lives towards adjustment.

Individuals with epilepsy can be seizure free with antiepileptic treatment, therefore they can have an acceptable quality of life enjoying a normal life.

I propose 'Metamyth'© as a psychological, creative, emotional and relational, support complementary to the medical for the treatment of epilepsy.

## The Poiesis of Metamyth©

The poiesis of "Metamyth"©, meaning, to make "Metamyth"©, I was inspired by philosophies and theories which I use as Therapeutic Elements in this therapy method. I mention here a few that I think will help as a background towards understanding the philosophy and practice of "Metamyth"©.

Aristotle the Greek philosopher [8], in his work Poetics, in a definition about the elements of good tragedy, speaks about 'catharsis'. It happened by producing the feelings of fear and pity in tragedy and laughter in comedy and through these feelings catharsis, and I will add, pleasure, and well being, or awareness of feelings and thoughts were experienced [8].

In "Metamyth"© of particular importance in working therapeutically with people with epilepsy is, the concept of catharsis, because it brings a release of tension and helps with social adjustment. Because epilepsy has a private as well as a public stigma, the collective aspect of catharsis has special importance. People with epilepsy inherit the historical burden of a scape-goated disease. Therefore for them personal cathartic release is vital for integration of personal identity free of such history [1].

Further release comes from movement [9] as well as relief by talking through and reflecting on the issues contained by the therapist.

In "Metamyth"© the therapist and the client act in the here and now, the reality of their own experiences and feelings. The use of role [10], if used, is intentional, helps to understand the different aspects of a client's identity in their life. By observing enactment of himself, or another person's character in the group, a client can find resemblances or come to an understanding about themselves.

"'Metamyth"© uses role and role distance at a deeper Jungian level by observing the concept of Archetypes [11]. Deeper psychological archetypal and emotional aspects are discovered. By performing the various roles the clients may generate new roles and allow themselves free from the pathological ones.

After a client has been involved in role activity it is necessary to derole in order to leave their enacted role and to relocate and readjust to their usual identities.

"Metamyth"© has as a purpose to stimulate the feelings with stories, and if possible, their enactment. Along with the story, the myth, between the client and the therapist is developing in the contained space of a "Metamyth"© session. *"It could be suggested that a mythology of healing is created between client and therapist which is enacted by their respective roles and is developing in the contained space of the therapeutic relationship and the dramatic material in the session"*[1].

"Metamyth'© is a holistic approach that includes mind, body, feeling and intuition into therapy as well as the culture where the patient comes from.

Although "Metamyth"© involves attention towards the inner world and expressing it symbolically it uses work with movement to help people with epilepsy free-up their body habits and introduce new possibilities.

In "Metamyth"© I aim to cultivate awareness of how the body functions and encourage trust in the mind- body interaction and expression of emotions. I believe that there is a psychological benefit of being grounded in the body. As an action therapy, it creates the opportunity for the client to experience the relationship that connects body emotion and identity [1].

Jung's idea of the persona refers to the role an individual plays in their public or social life which can mask other aspects of personality [12]. This idea is particularly important when working with people with epilepsy due to their own fragile persona or self-image." Metamyth"© can help in recognizing the hidden side and support the process of building a conscious link to the unconscious or the neglected aspects of the personality [13]. This can perhaps enable them to accept their true identity and feel a greater sense of wholeness.

Sometimes it might be difficult to reach the inner world of people who have epilepsy because they are used to keep their condition secret. The ritual in our work offers the possibility to access the inner world. It is a way to develop familiarity with the work and the people involved.

Play is important because it is a developmental activity through which human beings explore. Winnicott's says: 'playing can be a form of communication in psychotherapy; and lastly psychoanalysis has been developed as a highly specialised form of playing in the service of communication with one self and others' [14]. "Metamyth"© work with people who have epilepsy is interested into bringing in the play, the past, and it also focuses into the spontaneity of the action and the creativity of the here and now.

"Metamyth"© offers people with epilepsy the chance to understand their condition and express it in their own words or paint it or dance it or sing it or sculpt it thus creating greater self-awareness and self-confidence.

As it is mentioned in the definition of "Metamyth"© this therapeutic method draws upon a neurobiological approach to Psychology and Therapy. I believe that the brain is an organ continually built and rebuilt by one's experiences. As I have described "Metamyth"© stimulates mind body intuition and personality. This creates meaningful and positive experiences that enhance change in relevant neural circuits and this is how and why "Metamyth"© therapy works. Theoretical perspectives and technological advances in brain imaging and recent research in intersecting the fields of neuroscience and psychotherapy support this [15, 16].

The 8 Elements mentioned above are also Tools and Means of "Metamyth"© Therapy which I incorporate into my clinical everyday work.

Some clients could not want to follow all these steps or find role play difficult in which case the therapist encourages them in the work that they want to do and respect their wishes and limitations.

Throughout as I have emphasised " therapist and client are creating an individual myth but one which is also full with unconscious collective, archetypal content which goes beyond the conscious intention of both" [17].

Much of my work in "Metamyth"© has to do with Mythology. It has to do with one's self in a great self-nourishing manner. Working with people who have epilepsy mythology can act as medium to help and support both internal and social processes.

*What "Metamyth"© is suggesting is a re-discovery and re-evaluation of what mythology has to offer in the modern and the post modern world"* [1].

'Metamyth'© as an art medium enables a heritage to the archetypal dimensions of the psyche which allows the instinctual and non-rational aspects of the self to become integrated with the cerebral and physiological.

It is usually the case that the physical body, is being looked after by medical science and the psychological issues also require being taken care of [13].

I suggest "Metamyth"© as an effective psychological therapy complementary to the medical treatment to address the inner life of aspects of the patients experience of epilepsy.

"Metamyth"© can be offered as a psychological treatment for people who have epilepsy as well as for any client population at any age, or any stage of development [13].

## An Example of "Metamyth"© Therapy in a Hospital

In the A University Clinic of Neurology and Psychiatry, Aeginition Hospital, Athens, Greece we have incorporated "Metamyth"© Dramatherapy as a psychological treatment for the people who have epilepsy in 2014.

Sessions take place parallel to the epilepsy clinic where the doctors neurologists/epileptologists, refer the patients who ask for psychological support to the "Metamyth"© clinic. We give the patients to read, a discription of this type of therapy and after they agree, they sign a consent form and make an appointment.

The patients within the age range of 22–80 years old, can be man and women, may have temporal lobe, idiopathic generalized, post traumatic, epilepsies, absences, or epilepsy with mental retardation, After the end of therapy the patients enter a follow up period of three months and an appointment to come back for a session. They are given a "Metamyth"© questionaire to fill in asking them how they feel having had this treatment. Results have shown that epilepsy patients acquire a lot of benefit, feel and even look healthier, during and after "Metamyth"© psychotherapy. In the evaluation methods I include their personal and their family's testimonies, the evaluation of the therapist [18] and that of their doctor.

People with psychogenic seizures or panic attacks find relief and calm, therefore the frequency of seizures decreases. There aren't many epilepsy patients who ask for emotional or psychological help. One of the reasons being, the sociocultural perception that they don't need it. The ones who do manage to access are empowered with confidence and learn to appreciate their skills and talents. Also it can help to come to a deeper understanding of their difficulties and to find the inner strength and will, to keep a good balance, and be positive in their attitude and approach. In my research I have not found reference in dramatherapy of people who have epilepsy andv I am pioneering this area of research with "Metamyth"©/Dramatherapy in the treatment of people who have epilepsy [1, 12].

Here are some quotes of what some of the patients have said:

"I enjoy that "Metamyth"© responds to my need to dream and to use my imagination".

"I have support to look for and bring back my talents".

"Helps me to define boundaries and encourages me when I make the right for me choices I take confidence".

"I was confused before I come to "Metamyth"© Therapy and now I feel things are one by one clearer inside. My problems also are clearer and I try to handle them step by step".

"I got what I wanted from "Metamyth"©Therapy, Confidence in myself and maturity. And when I am with other people I have a good time".

"I feel independent and I complain less because that is something that I don't like in myself anymore".

"I remember sessions where I found solutions for important issues in my life".

"Metamyth"© made me see my problems from another perspective and to be more in peace. The symptoms of my condition are milder now".

"Metamyth"© helped me put an order inside. I feel peaceful even when I have symptoms".

"I gained confidence".

"In comparison with other psychotherapies "Metamyth"© is more pleasant".

"From my therapist I took support, every moment, strength, devotion, courage, love".

"My relationship with the therapist was one of trust, inspiration , exclusivity, support, love".

"I take calmness with me as I go away from my session".

"I gained confidence, integrity, joy, maturity".

"Metamyth"© is a suitable psychological approach for people who have epilepsy because it provides the opportunity to explore identity, offers possibilities for emotional expression and release. It helps to develop coping mechanisms arising from the sudden occurrences of seizures, addresses social and personal stigmata attached to these occurrences and provides an empowering approach.

## End Note

"Metamyth"©/Dramatherapy is an important psychotherapeutic method for people with epilepsy.

## References

1. Valeta T. The potential of dramatherapy in the treatment of epilepsy. MA thesis, University of Derby; 2009.
2. Valeta T. "Metamyth"© and its application in everyday life. Lecture neurolinguistic programming course. London: Regents College; 2000.
3. Kanner AM. Depression in epilepsy: a complex relation with unexpected consequences. Curr Opin Neurol. 2008;21:190–4.
4. Engel J Jr, Pentley TA, editors. Epilepsy a comprehensive textbook. 2nd ed. Philladelphia: Lippincott William & Wilkins; 2008.
5. Freud S (orig.1928) An autobiographical study, inhibitions, symptoms and anxiety, lay analysis, and other works, vol. 5. London: Vintage; 2001.
6. Jacoby A, Austin JK. Social stigma for adults and children with epilepsy. Epilepsia. 2007;48(Suppl 9):6–9.
7. Arnston P, et al. The perceived psychosocial consequences of having epilepsy. In: Whitman S, Herman B, editors. Psychopathology in epilepsy: social dimentions. Oxford: Oxford University Press; 1986.
8. Aristotle. Poetics. trans. Vellacott Ph. London: Harvard University Press; 1995.
9. Chodorow J. Dance therapy and depth psychology. New York: Routledge; 2005.
10. Chodorow J. Dramatherapy: concepts, theories and practices. 2nd ed. Sprinfield: Charles C Thomas; 1994.
11. Jung CJ. Memories, dreams, reflections. London: Fontana Press; 1995.

12. Jung C. The collected works, vol. 13. London: Routledge and Keggan Paul; 1954.
13. Valeta T. "Metamyth" © and Dramatherapy: an innovative approach for people with epilepsy. In: Schrader C, editor. Ritual theatre the power of dramatic ritual in personal development groups and clinical practice. London: Jessica Kingsley; 2012. p. 275–90.
14. Winnicott DW. Playing and reality. New York: Routledge; 2005.
15. Damazio AR. The feeling of what happens. New York: Harcourt Brace; 1999.
16. Siegel DJ. Developing mind: toward a neurobiology of interpersonal experience. New York: Guilford; 1999.
17. Hillman J. Archetypal psychology. Putnam: Spring; 2004.
18. Jennings S. The handbook of dramatherapy. London: Routledge; 2008.

# Complementary and Alternative Treatments for Epilepsy

**20**

## Abstract

Complementary and alternative treatments are a group of diverse health care systems, practices, and products that are not generally considered part of conventional medicine. These treatments are usually in addition (complementary) or instead (alternative) to main-stream medical therapy Their use has increased over the past two decades, and surveys have shown that up to 44% of patients with epilepsy are using some form of such treatments. A significant problem with them is that their safety and effectiveness is not tested with well-designed scientific studies. Some may be very helpful and harmless, but others may interfere with the medically prescribed drugs, weaken their effectiveness or cause side effects. Complementary therapy organisations can provide names of registered therapists, and advice about what to look for in a good therapist.

## Keywords

Relaxation techniques • Meditation • Yoga • Biofeedback • Nutritional supplements • Herbal supplements • Chiropractic care • Magnet therapy • Prayers • Acupuncture • Reiki • Homeopathy • Physical exercise programs • Aroma therapy • Biofeedback

## What Is Complementary and Alternative Medicine (CAM)?

Patients and health care practitioners often use other than conventional medical treatments in order to improve seizure control, to reduce side effects and/or to improve comorbidities and quality of life. These treatments are usually in addition (complementary) or instead (alternative) to main-stream medical therapy. Another

© Springer International Publishing AG 2017
T. Valeta, *The Epilepsy Book: A Companion for Patients*,
DOI 10.1007/978-3-319-61679-7_20

137

term is "integrative medicine" to emphasize that both types of treatment (conventional and complementary) are combined (integrated) in the patient's care.

CAM is a common short name for complementary and alternative medicine. Therapies listed as CAM are generally the same ones indicated by the term "alternative therapies." The difference lies in whether the person also uses conventional therapies.

CAM is defined by the American National Centre of Complementary and Alternative Medicine as a group of diverse medical and health care systems, practices, and products that are not generally considered part of conventional medicine and are not generally taught at the western medical colleges.

The use of CAM has increased over the past two decades, and surveys have shown that up to 44% of patients with epilepsy are using some form of CAM treatment. Conventional health professionals are becoming more interested in these treatments.

Some CAM therapies have long histories in some countries, cultures and traditions and some are recent developments. In epilepsy, for instance, the ketogenic diet began as an alternative therapy but has been scientifically tested and is rapidly being accepted as a conventional therapy for certain types of epilepsy (see Chap. 21 on Dietary treatments for epilepsy and Ketogenic diet). Some people around the world do not have access to modern drug regimens; which is why patients choose CAM, as they are easily accessible.

## What Are the Benefits and the Risks of CAM?

As with any treatment, it is important to consider safety before using complementary health products and practices. Safety depends on the specific therapy, and each complementary product or practice should be considered on its own.

Mind and body practices such as meditation and yoga, for example, are generally considered to be safe in healthy people when practiced appropriately. Natural products such as herbal medicines or botanicals are often sold as dietary supplements and are readily available to consumers; however, there is a lot we don't know about the safety of many of these products, in part because a manufacturer does not have to prove the safety and effectiveness of a dietary supplement before it is available to the public (see Chap. 21 on Dietary treatments for epilepsy and Ketogenic diet). Two of the main safety concerns for dietary supplements are:

- The possibilities of drug interactions—for example, research has shown that St. John's wort interacts with drugs in ways that can interfere with their intended effects.
- The possibilities of product contamination—supplements have been found to contain hidden prescription drugs or other compounds, particularly in dietary supplements marketed for weight loss, sexual health including erectile dysfunction, and athletic performance or body-building.

A significant problem with CAM is that their safety and effectiveness is not tested with well-designed scientific studies. Some of them may be very helpful and harmless, but others may interfere with the medically prescribed drugs, weaken their effectiveness or cause side effects.

There is no firm scientific evidence to suggest that any type of CAM can effectively treat epilepsy. Some complementary therapies may reduce epileptic seizures indirectly because they make you feel better generally. If stress is a trigger for your seizures, a therapy that helps you to feel less stressed may help you to have fewer seizures. However, some complementary therapies can increase the risk of seizures, so it is important to know as much as possible about your own epilepsy, and the therapies you receive. Patients should continue taking antiepileptic drugs, even when using complementary treatments. These matters should be openly discussed with the treating physician or epilepsy specialist nurse.

## What Should I Do If I Decide to Use CAM for My Epilepsy?

If you decide to use CAM make sure that this is through qualified and registered CAM therapists and tell them about your epilepsy, your seizures, any other conditions you have and any medication that you take. Complementary therapy organisations can provide names of registered therapists, and advice about what to look for in a good therapist:

1. Ask for credentials. Seek a licensed practitioner who has trained at an accredited school.
2. Ask how much experience the practitioner has in general and treating epilepsy in particular

Look up product or practice and safety information—including side effects and cautions—on the list provided in the National Center for Complementary and Alternative Medicine (NCCAM) fact sheets, MedlinePlus, or other relevant websites.

In the United States the formal agency working in this area is the National Center for Complementary and Alternative Medicine, which is part of the National Institutes of Health. The NCCAM website is a reliable source of up-to-date information and links to other resources: http://nccam.nih.gov/

http://epilepsy.med.nyu.edu/diagnosis-treatment/alternative-therapies
http://www.epilepsysociety.org.uk/complementary-therapies#.UjLfJ8aKKSp.
http://www.ice-epilepsy.org/alternative-therapy.html
http://www.annalsofian.org/article.asp?issn=0972-2327;year=2011;volume=14;issue=3;spage=148;epage=152;aulast=Saxena
http://reference.medscape.com/medline/abstract/16822357
http://en.wikipedia.org/wiki/Alternative_medicine
See also the book "Complementary and Alternative Therapies for Epilepsy" by O. Devinsky, S. C. Schachter, S. V. Pacia; Demos Medical Publishing 2012.

## What Are the Main CAM Used in Epilepsy and How They Work?

The two broad areas—natural products and mind and body practices—capture most complementary health approaches. However, some approaches may not neatly fit into either of these groups—for example, the practices of traditional healers, Ayurvedic medicine from India, traditional Chinese medicine, homeopathy, and naturopathy.

There are various CAM modalities used by patients with epilepsy and these include: various relaxation techniques, meditation, yoga, biofeedback, nutritional and herbal supplements, dietary measures, chiropractic care, magnet therapy, prayers, acupuncture, Reiki, and homeopathy, fish oil supplementation, traditional Chinese medications and physical exercise programs [1–6]. The most commonly cited CAMs included acupuncture, botanical/herbals, chiropractic care, magnet therapy, prayers, stress management, and yoga.

Three Cochrane reviews highlighted that based on observational data, there appears to be a beneficial effect on seizure frequency related to yoga, stress management (aroma therapy, desensitization, relaxation, biofeedback, massage, and acupuncture) or acupuncture but there is no firm scientific evidence to support the use of any of these treatments. Therefore, the evidence to encourage any of these therapies is speculative at best. However, stress management and other nonmedicinal CAM that help to reduce stress are likely to be beneficial when used with conventional epilepsy treatments [3–6].

## Relaxation Therapies

Relaxation therapy involves a variety of strategies to reduce stress and foster relaxation. Biofeedback, massage and aromatherapy, breathing manoeuvres, hypnosis, meditation, and other techniques can be employed.

**Biofeedback** has been shown to help people with high blood pressure, migraine headaches, and pain. Researchers have investigated whether biofeedback can help control seizures, but the results have not been encouraging. However, patients who have seizures triggered by anxiety or stressful situations may benefit from this therapy, in addition to their seizure medications.

**Massage** is often used to reduce tension and pain in muscles, help with poor sleep patterns, improve relaxation and reduce stress. All types of massage can be carried out with or without oil, and can involve the use of aromatherapy oils. However, these oils should only be used by a qualified aromatherapist who is trained to know which oils are safe for use in epilepsy.

**Physical exercise programs** can exert beneficial actions such as reduction of seizure susceptibility, reduction of anxiety and depression, and consequently, improvement of quality of life of individuals with epilepsy, exercise can be a potential candidate as non-pharmacological treatment of epilepsy.

**Yoga** is a safe and effective way to increase physical activity, especially strength, flexibility and balance. There is some evidence that regular yoga practice is beneficial for people with high blood pressure, heart disease, aches and pains – including lower back pain – depression and stress. For the treatment of epilepsy, the physical discipline of yoga seeks to re-establish a balance (union) between those aspects of a person's health that cause seizures.

## Acupuncture

Although there has been no evidence that acupuncture can directly improve epilepsy, it has been found to be effective in reducing stress and anxiety, which may then result in less seizures for some people with epilepsy. It can also improve wellbeing and underlying health, and help with headaches or fatigue associated with seizures. Many general physicians' surgeries are now making acupuncture available to patients through the NHS.

For more information about acupuncture contact the British Acupuncture Council (BAcC) at http://www.acupuncture.org.uk/

## Autogenic Training

Autogenic therapy is a self-generated therapy for mind and body. It comprises several strands, the main element of which is autogenic training.

There have been no specific studies of autogenic training in relation to epilepsy. However, some people who use this therapy report having better emotional balance, coping ability, wellbeing, quality of sleep, ability to relax, confidence and energy. They also report decreased anxiety, irritability and reactions to stress.

See British Autogenic Society at: http://www.autogenic-therapy.org.uk/

## Homeopathy

Homeopathy involves treating the individual with highly diluted substances, given mainly in tablet form, with the aim of triggering the body's natural system of healing. Homeopathy is based on the principle that you can treat 'like with like', that is, a substance which causes symptoms when taken in large doses, can be used in small amounts to treat those same symptoms. Homeopathic medicines (which homeopaths call remedies) are prepared by specialist pharmacies using a careful process of dilution and succussion (a specific form of vigorous shaking). Although there is no evidence that homeopathic treatments directly help epilepsy, some patients feel better and more in control of their epilepsy.

For more information visit the Royal London Hospital for Integrated Medicine (http://www.uclh.nhs.uk/OurServices/OurHospitals/RLHIM/Pages/Home.aspx) or the British Homeopathic Association (http://www.britishhomeopathic.org/).

## References

1. Devinsky O, Schachter SC, Pacia SV. Complementary and alternative therapies for epilepsy. New York: Demos Medical Publishing; 2012.
2. Sirven JI. Complimentary and alternative medicine for epilepsy. In: Panayiotopoulos CP, editor. Atlas of epilepsies. London: Springer; 2010. p. 1697–9.
3. Hartmann N, Neininger MP, Bernhard MK, Syrbe S, Nickel P, Merkenschlager A, et al. Use of complementary and alternative medicine (CAM) by parents in their children and adolescents with epilepsy—prevelance, predictors and parents' assessment. Eur J Paediatr Neurol. 2016;20:11–9.
4. McConnell BV, Applegate M, Keniston A, Kluger B, Maa EH. Use of complementary and alternative medicine in an urban county hospital epilepsy clinic. Epilepsy Behav. 2014;34:73–6.
5. Doering JH, Reuner G, Kadish NE, Pietz J, Schubert-Bast S. Pattern and predictors of complementary and alternative medicine (CAM) use among pediatric patients with epilepsy. Epilepsy Behav. 2013;29:41–6.
6. Ricotti V, Delanty N. Use of complementary and alternative medicine in epilepsy. Curr Neurol Neurosci Rep. 2006;6:347–53.

# Dietary Treatments for Epilepsy and Ketogenic Diet

**21**

## Abstract

A balanced diet is recommended for every person in order to keep healthy and active. However, there is little evidence that a balanced diet has a direct effect on seizures. Also, there is currently no evidence that any type of food consistently triggers seizures in people with epilepsy. Nearly 20% of patients who take prescription antiepileptic drugs also take herbal supplements. Unlike drugs, herbal therapies are classified by the Food and Drug Administration as dietary supplements and are not subject to regulations concerning their preparation, safety, or effectiveness. These items can both be of significant concern and/or promise because they may potentially be efficacious or dangerous either by a direct proconvulsant (induce seizures) effect or by interacting with ongoing antiepileptic drug treatment. Dietary treatments such as ketogenic diet can help some people with poorly controlled seizures by using specific levels of fat, carbohydrate and protein. The ketogenic diet has been shown to be particularly helpful for some epilepsy conditions such as epileptic encephalopathies. Several studies have shown that the ketogenic diet does reduce or prevent seizures in many children whose seizures could not be controlled by medications.

## Keywords

Herbals • Botanicals • Balanced diet • Modified Atkins diet • Intractable epilepsy • Epileptic encephalopathies

© Springer International Publishing AG 2017
T. Valeta, *The Epilepsy Book: A Companion for Patients*,
DOI 10.1007/978-3-319-61679-7_21

## Can Any Special Diet Help Prevent Seizures?

A balanced diet is recommended for every person in order to keep healthy and active. However, there is little evidence that a balanced diet has a direct effect on seizures. A balanced diet is generally made up of carbohydrates, fats, proteins, vegetables and fruit, and drinking plenty of fluids.

**Carbohydrates** include sugar, starch and fibre. They are found in potatoes, bread, pasta and rice. They are the main source of energy. Wholegrain versions of foods containing carbohydrates provide extra vitamins, minerals and fibre (which helps to remove waste from the body).

**Fats** include oils, oily fish, nuts and seeds. Fats help us to absorb nutrients including some important vitamins, and keep us warm. They help keep our cells healthy and give us energy.

**Proteins** are in dairy foods such as milk and cheese, and also in meat, fish, beans, lentils and eggs. They are essential for the body to develop and repair itself, they build and support our muscles, hormones, enzymes, red blood cells and immune system.

**Vegetables and fruit** of various colours provide vitamins and minerals. They also help protect us from infection, damage to our cells and diseases. Currently it is recommended that we should eat at least five portions of vegetables or fruit per day (one portion is roughly a handful).

Cooked food is usually healthier when steamed, baked, grilled, poached or boiled, rather than fried.

## Can Any Food Trigger Seizures?

There is currently no evidence that any type of food consistently triggers seizures in people with epilepsy. Some people with epilepsy avoid certain foods if they seem to trigger seizures and some avoid food with colourings and preservatives, monosodium glutamate or artificial sweeteners. Many foods labelled 'low-fat' contain these artificial ingredients. Grapefruit juice and pomegranate juice do not trigger seizures, but they can make the side effects of some antiepileptic drugs (including carbamazepine) more likely. See: https://www.epilepsysociety.org.uk/diet-and-nutrition#. WH_BRvmLTIU

## What Herbals and Botanicals Are Used for Epilepsy?

Nearly 20% of patients who take prescription drugs also take herbal supplements. Unlike drugs, herbal therapies are classified by the Food and Drug Administration as dietary supplements and are not subject to regulations concerning their preparation, safety, or effectiveness. These items can both be of significant concern and/or promise because they may potentially be efficacious or dangerous either by a direct pro-convulsant (induce seizures) effect or by interacting with ongoing anti-epileptic drug treatment.

Cases have been reported of herbal medicines for epilepsy containing antiepileptic drugs such as phenobarbital. Other ethical concerns include the use of animal products in some herbal medicines. Always consult your current doctor before taking herbal medicines, whether prescribed or 'over the counter'.

Herbal therapies are prepared from the flowers, leaves, stems, bark, or roots of plants. Some of these can be taken directly, but others undergo various forms of processing, such as drying of bark.

Herbal therapy is ancient, dating back to prehistoric times. Some modern drugs are derived from plants of herbal therapy. Texts from the eighteenth and nineteenth centuries describe many herbal therapies for epilepsy, including mistletoe, foxglove (digitalis), and cannabis sativa (marijuana), but few were found to be of much help. The herbal medicines that are alleged, but not proven, to have a beneficial effect on seizures include:

- Ailanthus altissima (Tree of Heaven)
- Artemisia vulgaris (mugwort)
- Calotropis procera (calotropis)
- Cannabis sativa (marijuana)
- Centella asiatica (hydrocotyle)
- Convallaria majalis (lily of the valley)
- Dictamnus albus (burning bush)
- Paeonia officinalis (peony)
- Scutellaria lateriflora (scullcap)
- Senecio vulgaris (groundsel)
- Taxus baccata (yew)
- Valeriana officinalis (valerian)
- Viscum album (mistletoe)

It appears that most patients perceive botanical therapies as somewhat beneficial but 43% of them also report an increase in their seizures.

The evidence about the use of cannabis (marijuana) to treat epilepsy has a long history with significant recent debates. A few high-profile cases in the US have led to the use of some chemicals derived from cannabis such as cannabidiol for the treatment of severe childhood epilepsies such as Dravet syndrome and Lennox-Gastaut syndrome. The early research results show that while some children appeared to improve after taking cannabidiol, others did not respond, or even worsened. Doctors say the findings underscore the need for more research on the extract. The laws in some states of America have even been changed to allow this.

http://www.epilepsy.com/learn/treating-seizures-and-epilepsy/other-treatment-approaches/medical-marijuana-and-epilepsy

## Are Herbal Therapies Safe?

Most of them are relatively safe in recommended doses, but adverse effects include rash, digestive disturbances, and headache. Overdoses can be dangerous and some natural herbs are deadly as for example hemlock (conium that killed Socrates), poisonous mushrooms and many others.

## Can Herbal Therapies Used Together with Antiepileptic Drugs?

Herbal therapies can interact with antiepileptic drugs. For example, St John's Wort can lower levels of certain antiepileptic drugs, including phenobarbital and phenytoin. Garlic may increase the levels of some antiepileptic drugs. Chamomile may intensify or prolong the effects of phenobarbital. Sedating herbs such as kava, valerian and passion flower can increase sedation produced by phenobarbital, benzodiazepines, and other drugs.

See also Chinese, Japanese, Indian and African herbal medicines in a very informative review on Herbal Remedies, Dietary supplements and Seizures which can be obtained in:

http://onlinelibrary.wiley.com/doi/10.1046/j.1528-1157.2003.19902.x/epdf
http://epilepsy.med.nyu.edu/diagnosis-treatment/alternative-therapies

## Are There Any Specific Dietary Treatments for Epilepsy?

Dietary treatments such as ketogenic diet can help some people with poorly controlled seizures by using specific levels of fat, carbohydrate and protein [1–7]. The modified Atkins diet and the low glycaemic index treatment are alternative, more relaxed, diets, which have been developed to try to overcome the restrictive nature of the ketogenic diets.

See details in.

https://www.charliefoundation.org/explore-ketogenic-diet/explore-1/introducing-the-diet

## What Is the Ketogenic Diet?

The ketogenic diet is a special high-fat, adequate in protein and low-carbohydrate diet that helps to control seizures in some people with epilepsy. It is prescribed by a physician and carefully monitored by a dietitian because it requires careful measurements of calories, fluids, and proteins.

The name ketogenic means that it produces ketones in the body (keto = ketone, genic = producing). Ketones are formed when the body uses fat for its source of energy. Usually the body uses carbohydrates (such as sugar, bread, pasta) for its fuel, but because the ketogenic diet is very low in carbohydrates, fats become the primary fuel instead.

In ketogenic-style diets, carbohydrates are restricted, and protein is provided only in amounts to meet the recommended dietary allowance to support growth and development. Fat is the main component of meals, providing roughly 90% of total calories. Meals are provided in exact portions with higher ratios of high-fat foods to encourage the breakdown of fat for energy. When the body has fewer calories from carbohydrates and protein, it switches from burning glucose to burning fat for energy.

## Who Is Likely to Benefit from the Ketogenic Diet?

The ketogenic diet has been shown to be particularly helpful for some epilepsy conditions such Dravet syndrome, Lennox-Gastaut syndrome, myoclonic-atonic epilepsy of Doose syndrome, Rett syndrome, tuberous sclerosis complex and infantile spasms. The ketogenic diet is a first-line treatment for the neurometabolic diseases glucose transporter type 1 (GLUT1) deficiency syndrome.

Several studies have shown that the ketogenic diet does reduce or prevent seizures in many children whose seizures could not be controlled by medications.

- Over half of children who go on the diet have at least a 50% reduction in the number of their seizures.
- Some children, usually 10–15%, even become seizure-free.

The diets are well-tolerated, but often discontinued because of their restrictiveness. In patients willing to try dietary treatment, the effect is seen quickly, giving patients the option whether to continue the treatment.

Recently, adults with epilepsy are one of the fastest growing groups of patients starting diets because of the assumption that outcomes are largely similar to children, with similar side effects.

## How a Patient Is Assessed and Why the Ketogenic Diet Is Administered?

Many factors must be considered, and the diet is not suitable for any patient with epilepsy. The strict diet should be implemented in specialized centres under close supervision and monitoring by doctors and dieticians experienced in this therapy. Under no circumstances should the diet be self- administered.

The primary reason for admission in most centres is to monitor for any increase in seizures or adverse side effects on the diet, ensure all medications are carbohydrate-free, and educate the families.

Referrals for the diet as a treatment for epilepsy are usually made by a paediatrician or paediatric neurologist.

## Are There Any Side Effects from the Ketogenic Diet?

The ketogenic diet is generally well tolerated and over 94% of patients have maintained appropriate growth parameters. A person starting the ketogenic diet may feel sluggish for a few days after the diet is started. Other short term problems include acidosis, exacerbation of gastrointestinal reflux, excessive ketosis, fatigue, food refusal, hypoglycaemia, increased seizure frequency.

Side effects that might occur if the person stays on the diet for a long time are:

- Kidney stones (5–8%)
- High cholesterol levels in the blood
- Dehydration
- Constipation
- Slowed growth or weight gain
- Reduced quantity of bone mass and bone fractures (requiring vitamin D supplementation)
- Gastritis and ulcerative colitis

Some antiepileptic drugs should be avoided when the patients are on ketogenic diet because their concentration may be altered and may cause toxicity. The diet may be lethal for patients with rare disorders such as pyruvate carboxylase deficiency.

Because the diet does not provide all the vitamins and minerals found in a balanced diet, the dietician will recommend vitamin and mineral supplements. The most important of these are calcium and vitamin D, iron, and folic acid.

## How Is the Patient Monitored over Time?

- Early on, the doctor will usually see the child every 1–3 months.
- Blood and urine tests are performed to make sure there are no medical problems.
- The height and weight are measured to see if growth has slowed down.
- As the child gains weight, the diet may need to be adjusted by the dietician.

## Can the Diet Ever Be Stopped?

If seizures have been well controlled for some time, usually 2 years, the doctor might suggest going off the diet.

- Usually, the patient is gradually taken off the diet over several months or even longer. Seizures may worsen if the ketogenic diet is stopped all at once.
- Children usually continue to take antiepileptic drugs after they go off the diet.
- In many situations, the diet has led to significant but not total, seizure control. Families may choose to remain on the ketogenic diet for many years in these situations.

## Where Can I Find Out More Information About the Diet?

The Charlie Foundation and Matthew's Friends are parent-run organizations for ketogenic diets.

See: https://www.charliefoundation.org/explore-ketogenic-diet/explore-1/introducing-the-diet

http://www.matthewsfriends.org/

Ketogenic News has been edited by Dr. Eric Kossoff, Medical Director of the John Hopkins Hospital Ketogenic Diet Program, one of the world experts on dietary treatment for epilepsy. KetoNews includes new information helpful for patients, parents, and caregivers who receive or provide diets for the treatment of epilepsy: http://www.epilepsy.com/learn/seizure-and-epilepsy-news/keto-news

Other than the internet, there are several books about the ketogenic diet available. One is The Ketogenic Diet: A Treatment for Children and Others with Epilepsy, by Drs. Freeman and Kossoff, which discusses the Johns Hopkins approach and experience.

## What Is the Modified Atkins Diet?

The Atkins diet is a low-carbohydrate diet used by some people in order to lose weight. The modified Atkins diet is a change of the "classic" ketogenic diet to make it less restrictive. Although the foods are very similar, there are key differences between the modified Atkins diet and the ketogenic diet.

- First, with the modified Atkins diet, there is no fluid or calorie restriction or limitation.
- Although fats are strongly encouraged, they are not weighed and measured. Most patients will consume plenty of dairy and oils.
- One of the biggest differences is that there are no restrictions on proteins. Typically 35% of calories for a patient on the modified Atkins diet come from protein.
- Foods are not weighed and measured, but carbohydrate counts are monitored by patients and/or parents.
- It is started outside of the hospital and the person does not need to fast before starting the diet.
- Lastly, foods can be eaten more freely in restaurants and outside the home, and families can do it as well.
- The diet is a "modified" Atkins diet as it allows for less carbohydrates than the traditional Atkins diet (15–20 g/day) and more strongly encourages fat intake. Please remember that no diet should be tried without a specialized neurologist involved.

Studies show the modified Atkins diet is very similar to the classic ketogenic diet in efficacy. It seems to help similar numbers of patients as the ketogenic diet (40–50% with greater than 50% seizure reduction, including approximately 15% seizure-free). It works for men and women equally and is being used actively in adolescents and adults. Like the ketogenic diet, it is mostly used for patients with daily seizures who have not fully responded to medications. It is under study for regions of the world with limited resources for which the classic ketogenic diet would be too difficult or time-consuming as well.

http://www.epilepsy.com/learn/treating-seizures-and-epilepsy/dietary-therapies/modified-atkins-diet

## Bibliography

1. Cross H. Epilepsy: behavioural, psychological, and ketogenic diet treatments. BMJ Clin Evid. 2015;2015
2. Felton EA, Cervenka MC. Dietary therapy is the best option for refractory nonsurgical epilepsy. Epilepsia. 2015;56:1325–9.
3. Klein P, Tyrlikova I, Mathews GC. Dietary treatment in adults with refractory epilepsy: a review. Neurology. 2014;83:1978–85.
4. Pasca L, De Giorgis V, Macasaet JA, Trentani C, Tagliabue A, Veggiotti P. The changing face of dietary therapy for epilepsy. Eur J Pediatr. 2016;175:1267–76.
5. Schoeler NE, Cross JH. Ketogenic dietary therapies in adults with epilepsy: a practical guide. Pract Neurol. 2016;16:208–14.
6. Stafstrom CE, Zupec-Kania B, Rho JM, editors. Ketogenic diet and related dietary treatments. Epilepsia. 2008;49(Suppl 8):1–133.
7. Vaccarezza MM, Silva WH. Dietary therapy is not the best option for refractory nonsurgical epilepsy. Epilepsia. 2015;56:1330–4.

# Safety in Epilepsy

# 22

**Abstract**

Keeping safe is important for everyone, whether or not they have epilepsy. Assessing the risks associated with the type and frequency of the seizures experienced and then implementing the necessary safety procedures are important steps in assuring personal safety and well-being. Safety recommendations are often common sense. Anything that affects a persown's conscious state, awareness or judgement can increase the risk of accidents. An Epilepsy Management/ Action Plan is a risk management tool that lets anyone, who has a person with epilepsy in their care, know what to do and what not to do when that person has a seizure.

**Keywords**

Swimming • Cycling • Leisure • Bathing • Driving • Occupational risks • Epilepsy action plan

## Keeping Safe Is Common Sense

Keeping safe is important for everyone, whether or not they have epilepsy.

Accidents can happen to anyone and everywhere in daily life. We take precautions and care to minimize these risks but we do not stop walking in the streets, cycling, driving, swimming, sporting, and socializing. We do not enclave ourselves in a fortified castle or a cage and the same should apply for people with epileptic seizures.

Common safety recommendations mainly refer to people with continuing epileptic seizures but again individual modifications are needed according to:

- The type of epileptic seizure (with or without loss of consciousness, with or without convulsions, with or without sufficient warning)
- The frequency of seizures
- Their predictability or not (reflex seizures, catamenial seizures)
- The likely time of their occurrence (in sleep, awakening, random)
- The presence of precipitating factors (fatigue, sleep deprivation, excessive alcohol consumption, flickering lights)

## Most of These Recommendations Are Common Sense

Knowing the type or types of seizure and epilepsy that a person has is important in risk assessment for their identification and prevention. Assessing the risks associated with the type and frequency of the seizures experienced and then implementing the necessary safety procedures are important steps in assuring personal safety and well-being. Therefore, these recommendations should be individualized. Matters that affect one person with epilepsy may be different and may not be an issue to those that affect others. For some people with epilepsy, their seizures pose a minimal risk of injury. For others, their seizures may require extra precaution to avoid injury. For example, seizures that occur without warning or those involving falls, loss of awareness, or postictal confusion after the seizure could result in injury.

Anything that affects a person's conscious state, awareness or judgement can increase the risk of accidents. Burns-related injuries are often reported in people who experience complex focal seizures and tonic-clonic seizures. Most common are injuries due to scalding in the kitchen or bathroom. Reducing hot water temperature can protect against burns. Similarly strategic placement of indoor heating appliances can minimize the risk of burns in the event of a tonic-clonic seizure.

Precautions in the home, workplace, educational settings, or while travelling or participating in activities may be necessary. New safety aids are continually being developed. High tech devices such as seizure-specific alarms triggered by seizure movements in bed, electronic tracking devices, and adapted showers that use infrared technology to shut off the water supply if a person falls.

**Leaflets with appropriate safety recommendations can be downloaded free from:**

http://www.epilepsy.org.uk/sites/epilepsy/files/epilepsyaction-booklet-safety.pdf
http://www.epilepsyscotland.org.uk/pdf/EpilepsyStayingSafe.pdf
http://www.epilepsymatters.com/english/pamphlets/safetyandepilepsy.pdf
http://www.epilepsyfoundation.org/resources/safety/index.cfm
http://www.manitobaepilepsy.org/pdf/safety.pdf
http://www.epilepsysociety.org.uk/Forprofessionals/Resourcesandtraining/Riskassessments
http://www.epilepsy.com/pdfs/transcripts_safety.pdf
http://www.epilepsyaustralia.net/Epilepsy_Information/Epilepsy_and_Risk/Epilepsy_and_Risk.aspx

## Assessment of Need and Epilepsy Risk Management

Local council social or volunteer services may be able to help by assessing the specific needs or carrying out a risk assessment.

Risk assessments are often carried out by an occupational therapist. They will provide information on what help, support or safety equipment might be needed because of epilepsy. The assessment can help to identify practical ideas for reducing risk to make situations safer.

Based on the medical assessment the occupational therapist will recommend amongst others guidelines in relation to driving, the use of dangerous machinery, working above ground level and high-risk activities such as scuba diving.

**An Epilepsy Management/Action Plan** is a risk management tool that lets anyone, who has a person with epilepsy in their care, know what to do and what not to do when that person has a seizure. Epilepsy Management Plans are often required by schools, pre-schools, child care centres, disability services, supported accommodation and respite services, and disability employment services. Plans help staff recognize seizure activity and provide documented procedures to follow should an emergency arise.

Plans should include the following information:

- Type of seizure/s
- Known triggers
- A description of the seizure pattern
- Who to contact in an emergency
- Name & dose of antiepileptic medication/s, and
- The time medication is administered.

Plans should also include step by step instructions from the treating doctor on

- How to manage the seizure and
- If emergency intervention treatment is required
- The specific circumstances under which it is to be administered, and
- The time-frame in which an ambulance should be called
- If the seizure activity requires emergency intervention, ensure that the medication is readily accessible. Bucchal midazolam is the intervention medication generally prescribed (see Chap. 16 on Profilactic Treatment with Antiepileptic Drugs)

## Check for Hazards Around You

Take a few moments to think about your home, work and leisure activities. Consider any risks that your seizures might create. Could you hurt yourself if you had a seizure? Is there a way that you could reduce the risk of harm to yourself or others?

There are many general safety strategies that you may not be using which would be useful. Do you have smoke alarms, fireguards, or power breakers fitted in your home? Is the hot water temperature controlled? Is your shower safe for anyone who falls, not just someone who has a seizure? Do you wear a bicycle helmet when riding?

Safety checklists are available from Epilepsy Affiliates and various community agencies:

https://www.epilepsy.org.au/sites/default/files/Seizure%20Smart%20-%20 Safety%20Checklist.pdf

https://www.epilepsyresearch.org.uk/wp-content/uploads/2014/04/epilepsy-checklist.pdf

http://www.epilepsyact.org.au/wp-content/uploads/2014/10/Safety-checklist.pdf

## Alarms

Smoke alarms are recommended for every household. This also applies for people with epilepsy who may also consider additional other types of alarms so as to inform others and get help when a seizure happens (particularly at night in sleep).

There are different types of alarm for different types of seizure. Some have a button to press for an impending seizure. Others are triggered by falls, convulsions, unusual noise, moisture. There is a wide range of bed alarms for infants and children with epilepsy (check with Disabled Living Foundation to find out which is suitable for your case). These can also detect bed occupancy (if the patient falls over or leaves the bed). Monitors can be personalized with the sensors required based on personal needs.

Small bells on to the bed or a baby intercom may also be used as they may alert for convulsions and noises during a seizure. Some parents find a video baby monitor (around £100 cost) more reassuring. Alarm systems are sometimes available through local social services departments or housing associations as part of an 'assessment of need'.

Carrying a pre-programmed cell phone or beeper is useful when in need.

If memory is affected, using a watch with an alarm, a day-timer, and a medication dispenser may be helpful.

## Safety at Home

Important and emergency telephone numbers are placed in an obvious place at every home and of course this should be re-enforced if a member of the family has epilepsy.

Consider the safety measures needed in a household with small children around. These are just a few points to consider. What happens in real life depends on individual circumstances which should be assessed carefully.

**In the house**
- Avoid hard and slipping flooring. Use if possible easily cleaned non-slip flooring, linoleum (lino), cushioned flooring or carpets.
- Avoid or protect staircases.
- Use protective covers on sharp corners of furniture, or have furniture with rounded edges.
- Use safety glass which is difficult to break or to hold together if it is broken. Safety glass film prevents glass shattering if it gets broken. This plastic film can be fitted onto glass doors and windows and is available from DIY and hardware stores and online suppliers.
- Do not leave hot appliances (e.g. stoves, irons) and open flames (e.g. fireplaces, candles) unprotected. Forced air heating is preferable to radiators, baseboards, and freestanding heaters. Cover radiators and hot pipes with radiators guards.
- Use appliances and tools with automatic shut-off switches.
- Use outdoor carpeting on concrete steps, porches, etc.


**In the kitchen and dining room**
- Preferably use microwave ovens; for conventional cookers use their back burners and fit them with a cooker guard in the front.
- Place pot handles facing to the back or the safe side of the cooker.
- Use cordless kettles that switch off automatically and also allow to pour the water than lifting the kettle.
- Use plastic rather than glass dishware; limit use of sharp knives and other utensils.
- Avoid carrying out pots or plates with boiling food, tea, milk, tea; serve hot liquids or food onto plates at the stove rather to the table; use a trolley to transfer hot food and liquids; use cups with lids.
- Grilling rather than frying food is safer.
- Place sharp utensils downwards in the dishwasher.
- Wear rubber gloves if washing glass or using sharp utensils.
- Keep frequently used items within easy reach to avoid having to climb up to high cupboards.
- Keep electrical appliances away from sinks.


**In the bedroom**
- Use low-level bed or mattresses; sleep in the middle of a large bed.
- Padded bed sides should be used with caution as one may become trapped in them.
- 'Anti-suffocation' pillows are available (see http://esuk.uk.com/index.php?option=com_content&view=article&id=6&Itemid=170).
- Use an alarm.

**In the bathroom**
- Take showers rather than baths; lower seat with a safety strap may be considered.
- Use a shower with a flat and anti-skidding floor; temperature monitor adjusting to a lower temperature; turn cold water on first and off last.
- Shower when someone else is home; keep bathroom doors open; doors should open outwards (or both ways).
- Mirrors and shower doors should be made from safety glass or plastic.
- An alarm monitor is useful.
- Turning on the cold tap first in the shower or basin and lowering the temperature of the hot water are good safety hints for any home.
- Avoid bathing in times and circumstances of increased risk of a seizures (see precipitating factors and juvenile myoclonic epilepsy).

## Gardening

Grass or bark chippings are a softer alternative to concrete or gravel and may reduce the risk of a severe injury if you fall.

Using a petrol lawn mower means there is less chance of cutting through the cable if you have a seizure. Some mowers will stop automatically when the handle is released. If you do use an electric mower a circuit breaker at the plug helps protect against electrocution.

If you have a pond, or you plan to build one, here are some safety tips that may be helpful.

- If possible put the pond where it can be seen from the house.
- A fence around large ponds can provide a safety barrier.
- Bushes or shrubs around the deeper side of a pond can stop you getting too close to the edge.
- It may be possible to fit a safety grid that sits just below the surface of the water. This can hold your weight if you fall on it, without spoiling the look of the pond.

## Outside Home

The risk of accidents and other unwanted outcomes from seizures such as having a seizure in the road, on public transport or at a special event, can be a source of fear for many people. With this in mind, being aware of the risks and taking reasonable steps to manage them, *people with epilepsy need not cut themselves off from the kinds of fulfilling lives they should be living. Many people with epilepsy lead full and active lives.*

Some people with epilepsy choose to wear or carry with them something that says they have epilepsy, in case of an accident. However this is a personal choice and does not appeal to everyone. Another option is to carry medical information in your wallet.

The UK Epilepsy Society produces a free 'I have epilepsy' card which you can write the type of seizures you have, what medication you are taking, and how you would like to be helped if you have a seizure. You can order your card from our online shop.

Other companies provide medical jewelry which can have your details on, address or a phone number where further information can be given. These can be helpful if you are taken to hospital as the doctors will be able to get information about your epilepsy and medication.

## Leisure Activities

Activities should not be restricted to the point where an individual cannot follow their interests or have some fun, however while seizures are not controlled some restrictions should be considered, particularly with those activities that carry greater risks. Ensure someone knows what you are doing.

Review the risks carefully before taking up sports that could put you or others in danger if you were suddenly unaware of what you are doing. Activities such as sky-diving, rock climbing, and scuba diving are restricted for people with seizures. Other activities which require special considerations are those that occur near or in water or heights. Always wear protective safety equipment during applicable activities, (such as helmets, floatation devices, and/or knee or elbow pads). Use the buddy system with certain exercise equipment and activities, such as hiking. When exercising, take frequent breaks, stay well-hydrated, and avoid over-exertion. Exercise on soft surfaces, such as grass, mats, or wood chips. If you are going to swim, make sure a lifeguard or someone who knows life saving techniques is present and knows that you have seizures. Use a lifejacket for watercraft activities.

### Swimming and water sports
- Never swim alone and while participating in water activities take a friend or carer with you
- Let a lifeguard know about your condition
- Wear lifejackets in boats and when fishing
- Avoid scuba diving and high board diving
- Avoid water that is too hot in spas and keep up fluids

### Cycling
- Always wear a helmet (this is law anyway)
- Use bike tracks/lanes where possible

### Generally
- Whenever participating in an activity where a fall may be possible or it poses the risk of a head injury, use protective head gear
- Be aware of over exertion or over heating
- Drink plenty of water
- If possible try to choose activities that take place on softer surfaces such as grass and mats

See details in:

https://www.epilepsy.org.uk/info/sports-leisure

https://www.epilepsysociety.org.uk/leisure-and-epilepsy

http://www.epilepsy.com/information/professionals/resource-library/links/recreation-and-leisure-activities

https://www.epilepsyresearch.org.uk/wp-content/uploads/2014/04/safetyandleisure.pdf

## Driving

There are laws about driving and epilepsy. In general people who have had a seizure are required to notify the licensing body and stop driving until a medical report is supplied. Most people can return safely to driving but the length of time a person must wait varies between individuals.

For people with epilepsy in the UK relevant questions and answers in regard to driving can be found in: https://www.epilepsy.org.uk/info/driving

This information covers the rules for holding a driving licence. And it explains how the agencies that issue driving licences work. It also tells you what help with transport costs is available, if you can't drive because of your epilepsy.

For people with epilepsy in USA relevant questions and answers in regard to driving can be found in: http://www.epilepsy.com/get-help/staying-safe/driving-and-transportation

To get a driver's license in most U.S. states, a person with epilepsy must be free of seizures that affect consciousness for a certain period of time. The seizure-free period varies from state to state. While some states still require a period of at least 1 year seizure free, most consider exceptions that would permit someone to drive after a shorter seizure-free interval (3–6 months).

Usually, the doctor who cares for the person with epilepsy must fill out a form stating the date of the last seizure, type and other relevant information. Some states ask for the doctor's recommendation about the person's ability to drive. In states that do not require a specific seizure-free period, the doctor's recommendation may carry considerable weight.

## Epilepsy and Work\Employment

Most people with epilepsy can work without worrying about safety issues. Some duties can often be made safer with a few changes. Employers are, in many cases, required by law to make such changes or accommodations. How you are affected by your seizures and your workplace setting will determine what safety considerations you may need. Review potential workplace hazards and which tasks are difficult as a result of the seizures and/or could trigger them. This can involve working amongst heights, heavy machinery, work time shifts or other conditions of the work place. As per workplace regulations, wear protective clothing and gear, such as gloves, safety glasses, boots, etc. when necessary. For details on specific questions see:

Epilepsy and Occupational Health—Epilepsy Scotland
www.epilepsyscotland.org.uk/pdf/ES-Occupational-Health-Guide.pdf
Work, employment and epilepsy|Epilepsy Society
https://www.epilepsysociety.org.uk/work-employment-and-epilepsy
Work and epilepsy|Epilepsy Action
https://www.epilepsy.org.uk/info/employment
Employment Help—What You Need to Know|Epilepsy Foundation
www.epilepsy.com/get...epilepsy/...epilepsy/employment-help-what-you-need-know
Work and epilepsy—employees|Epilepsy Action
https://www.epilepsy.org.uk/info/employment/legal-matters
Employers—information on employing a person with epilepsy
https://www.epilepsysociety.org.uk/employers-information-employing-person-epilepsy
What jobs can I do with epilepsy?|Epilepsy Society
https://www.epilepsysociety.org.uk/what-jobs-can-i-do-epilepsy
Telling your employer about your epilepsy|Epilepsy Society
https://www.epilepsysociety.org.uk/telling-your-employer-about-your-epilepsy
Epilepsy and employment—Wikipedia, the free encyclopedia
https://en.wikipedia.org/wiki/Epilepsy_and_employment

## Parents with Epilepsy Caring for Children

Like all parents and caregivers, childproof your home as much as possible. Use safety gates near stairs. You could move a baby in a stroller around the house if you think it is necessary. Dress, change, and sponge bathe a baby on the floor or in the bed, using a changing pad. Do not bathe a baby when you are alone. Tell children what to do during a seizure and when and how to call for help.

Tips for looking after a baby or young child when you have epilepsy can be found in: https://www.epilepsy.org.uk/info/caring-children

# Psychosocial Impact of Epilepsy

# 23

**Abstract**

Epilepsy is associated with significant neurobiological, cognitive, psychological, and social problems.

The psychosocial impact of epilepsy is multitude with numerous and often complex synergistically interacting medical, psychological, economic, educational, personal, and social repercussions. It depends on several factors: severity of epilepsy; neurological dysfunction; complexity of clinical management and side effects of antiepileptic drugs; family environment; perception of the disorder; restrictions in the activities; the level of health care and social support, and the extent of resources available to deal with the epilepsy. Recently, there are several well organized collaborative efforts to improve care and minimize the psychosocial impact of epilepsy.

**Keywords**

Epilepsy psychopathology • Newly diagnosed epilepsy • Children with epilepsy • Women with epilepsy • Elderly with epilepsy • Atlas of epilepsy • Stigma

## The Psychosocial Impact of Epilepsy Is Severe

The diagnosis and management of epilepsy has made significant progress in recent years. The diagnosis has become more specific with the recognition of epileptic syndromes and diseases. The management has extended beyond the treatment of epileptic seizures to deal with a number of psychosocial issues that affect the quality of life of patient and family. These changes are now well reflected in the new definition of epilepsies by the International League Against

Epilepsy (ILAE), which has been broadened to include the neurobiological, cognitive, psychological, and social consequences: "epilepsy is a disorder of the brain characterized by an enduring predisposition to generate epileptic seizures and by the neurobiological, cognitive, psychological, and social consequences of this condition" [1].

The psychosocial impact of epilepsy on adults, children and family is multitude with numerous and often complex synergistically interacting medical, psychological, economic, educational, personal, and social repercussions [2–5]. It depends on several factors: severity of epilepsy; neurological dysfunction; complexity of clinical management and side effects of antiepileptic drugs; family environment; perception of the disorder by the child, family, and society; restrictions in the activities as well as innate coping abilities of the child and family; the level of health care and social support, and the extent of resources available to deal with the epilepsy [6].

Some research shows that children with epilepsy, even those with new-onset seizures, are at increased risk of psychopathology. They are up to 4.7 times more likely to have behavioral problems than healthy children; such problems are thought to be already present in the earliest stage of the disease, even in children with "epilepsy only". A meta-analysis of 46 relevant studies found that attention, thought, and social problems were relatively specific to epilepsy, whereas problems with withdrawal, somatic complaints, anxiety/depression, delinquency, and aggression were not significantly different to those of healthy siblings or children with other chronic diseases [7]. The proportion of children with behavioral problems is lower in patients with new-onset epilepsy than in patients with chronic epilepsy. Comparisons with siblings suggest that psychopathology in children with epilepsy may be associated with family factors, especially where behavioral disorders appear to be more generic.

Parents are integral to the functioning and quality of life of their children and, therefore, the health-related quality of life of a child largely depend on the parents' attitudes, reactions, education and adjustment, and the support they may have. The attitudes, fears, wishes, and the multidisciplinary support needed by parents of children with epilepsy are immense. The impact of epilepsy on the patient's family largely depends on the role of the affected member (e.g., mother, father, siblings, spouses, or other carers). Compared to control groups, families with a child with epilepsy generally score worse on the whole range of family factors and these in return adversely influence the psychopathology of children with epilepsy [8].

The impact of children's epilepsies and the resulting parenting needs are even greater for mothers whose traditional primary role, in most societies, is raising of their children. In many societies, women are mainly involved in domestic tasks and child care or enter low-paid employment out of economic necessity. In developed countries, women are more career and education oriented. Mothers sustain a greater burden of care exhibit higher levels of strain and show higher levels of anxiety for the future and academic achievement of their children, than fathers [9].

## The Psychosocial Impact of Newly Identified Epileptic Seizures

A first epileptic seizure is a sudden, unexpected, and often devastating life event. The incident generates a cascade of concerns about the cause of the seizure, its effect on the brain, the possibility of recurrence, when and where it might recur, and whether this is the start of a developing underlying disorder of uncertain severity and aetiology. These concerns are accompanied by significant personal and family lifestyle changes, including psychological and suicidal behavioural, social, and financial effects that can be immense.

Cognitive and behavioural problems in children with newly diagnosed seizures have been documented:

- Behavioural problems may be present at or before the onset of seizures and therefore cannot be attributed solely to poor adjustment to living with a chronic condition.
- Children who developed recurrent seizures had significantly higher total and internalizing behavioural problem scores compared with healthy siblings and children without recurrent seizures.
- Children who had recurrent seizures were significantly more likely to be in the at-risk range for attention problems than children without recurrent seizures.

Other factors significantly associated with behavioural problems in addition to recurrent seizures are male gender, lower caregiver education, and older age of the child at seizure onset. There also was a trend for behaviour-problem scores to be higher when children were treated with an AED. The authors concluded that seizures, medication, and psychosocial factors contribute to these behavioural problems.

## The Psychosocial Impact of Established Long-Term Epilepsy

Additional information and long-term multidisciplinary support is needed for parents with children who have long-term epilepsy, which entails recurrent seizures for a variable length of time that may be lifelong. These parents have to prepare themselves for their children's continuing medical care of a chronic disease and its consequences, combined with the limitations that the seizures themselves impose on their physical, educational, financial, vocational, social, and subsequent marital state.

Parents of children with enduring long-term epilepsy often find themselves alone in dealing with delays to diagnosis, gaining access to specialists and proper management, encountering restrictions at school, and navigating through complicated health care, educational, and social services systems without guidance. Facing all of these situations, parental anxiety increases and parents themselves suffer a diminished quality of life. Parents also desperately need information about how to facilitate the transition from school to employment, how to maximize their child's academic achievement, and how to improve their child's mood.

## Febrile Seizures and Benign Childhood Epilepsy

Reactions, concerns, and needs are also eminent in parents of children with febrile and benign childhood seizures, although they are more fortunate with regard to prognosis, current and future prospects, and responsibilities than those of other epilepsies. These seizures are often severe and contrast with the physician's perception that they are simple and benign conditions [10].

See details in the Chap. 24 on Psychosocial Aspects, Parental Reactions and Needs in Idiopathic Focal Epilepsies.

## Women and Epilepsy

Women with epilepsy face special challenges in many biological and psychosocial aspects that are different from men [11]. The biological areas affected by epilepsy and AEDs include the menstrual cycle from menarche to menopause, sexuality and contraception, fertility, pregnancy and breastfeeding. Maternal parenting may become handicapped by safety issues of continuing epileptic seizures and adverse AED effects. The psychosocial, safety and legal issues are also of paramount importance in women with epilepsies who take care of children, partners or parents.

See details in the Chap. 12 on Women and Epilepsy.

## Elderly and Epilepsy

In the elderly, the incidence of new onset epileptic seizures dramatically increases to about 7–8%. People in this age group often have to adopt a different lifestyle to the one they had previously [12].

The elderly may also have to deal with age-related disorders such as cerebrovascular disease, Alzheimer disease and other causes of dementia. They may have to take several medications, and their metabolism, sensitivity and response to AEDs differs from that in younger adults; co-medication with other drugs is often problematic. Declining memory and intellectual function may also lead to poor compliance.

Old age is associated with an increased risk for osteoporosis and fractures, which may be made worse in those with epilepsy by falls, effects of enzyme-inducing antiepileptic drug on vitamin D and unsteadiness.

## Recommendations

The problems and continued need for information and support of patients with newly diagnosed epilepsy have been well documented. Conveying the diagnosis of "epilepsy" to a patient is a difficult and complex task that a physician has to do within a 30–45-min consultation. Yet, this is a crucial time to establish a strong relationship between patient and health care professional [13].

When an incontrovertible diagnosis of epileptic seizures has been reached, it is crucial that patients or parents are given sufficient time and opportunity to discuss their concerns with the medical specialists, who should provide:

- An accurate diagnosis, including precise cause, risk of recurrence, prognosis, type of management, possible hereditary factors, and adverse effects of treatment
- An assessment of the immediate and future effects of epilepsy on the physical, mental, behavioural, educational, family, social, and vocational aspects of the patient's life
- Information about preventing injury in leisure and other activities
- Information about possible avoidance measures' (e.g., reflex epilepsies and precipitating factors) and early recognition of the onset of an impending major epileptic attack (e.g., myoclonic jerks and absences), including means of terminating a seizure, particularly if it is lengthy and life-threatening

Comprehensive and well-structured first seizure clinics should be widely established so as to offer patients the best possible health care and psychosocial support at this early stage.

## Improving Care

The ILAE has been working with the International Bureau for Epilepsy and the WHO to form the Global Campaign against Epilepsy. This campaign has completed several demonstration projects and new ventures are in place to improve care in regions with limited resources, to establish regional atlases of epilepsy resources by country, legislation, and to carry out collaborative studies involving developing and developed countries. A document entitled "Out of the Shadows" has also been published [14].

Simultaneously, the National Institutes of Health and the National Institute of Neurological Disorders and Stroke in the USA, and members of the Epilepsy Community worldwide have developed a plan of action that describes specific benchmarks that can be reached within the next few years to improve the life of people with epilepsies. A prominent benchmark is to identify and prevent comorbidities of epilepsy, such as cognitive and memory dysfunction, depression, anxiety, attention disorders, autistic features, language disturbances, learning disabilities, and sleep disturbances among others. This can be achieved by a competent health care system involving all health care professionals including physicians, specialist nurses, psychologists, psychotherapists, and pharmacists. Educating parents and their families through seminars, courses, and lectures is essential in order to reduce anxiety, panic, and psychosocial morbidity in those affected. Child-centred, family focused counseling models for parents are used to help them deal with their anger, resentment, grief, and anxiety, and thus contribute to effective child care. Stigma has profound effects on social identity, discrimination, and overall quality of life for parents and patients with seizures, even for the benign types. See Chap. 25 on Stigma and how to combat it. I Encourage psychological therapies for patients and family and especially "Metamyth"© the psychological therapy for the people who have epilepsy. See Chap. 19.

Together these initiatives aim to improve the life of all patients with epilepsy, regardless of age and sex, and to enable patients and their families to think positively and to be significant contributors to our society.

## References

1. Fisher RS, van Emde BW, Blume W, Elger C, Genton P, Lee P, et al. Epileptic seizures and epilepsy: definitions proposed by the International League Against Epilepsy (ILAE) and the International Bureau for Epilepsy (IBE). Epilepsia. 2005;46:470–2.
2. Hermann B, Jacoby A. The psychosocial impact of epilepsy in adults. Epilepsy Behav. 2009;15(Suppl 1):S11–6.
3. Camfield PR. Problems for people with epilepsy beyond seizures. Epilepsia. 2007;48(Suppl 9):1–2.
4. Sillanpaa M, Cross HJ. The psychosocial impact of epilepsy in childhood. Epilepsy Behav. 2009;15(Suppl 1):S5–10.
5. Quintas R, Raggi A, Giovannetti AM, Pagani M, Sabariego C, Cieza A, et al. Psychosocial difficulties in people with epilepsy: a systematic review of literature from 2005 until 2010. Epilepsy Behav. 2012;25:60–7.
6. The psychosocial burden of epilepsy: ameliorating the impact. Proceedings of a workshop, 2008, Oxford, UK. Epilepsy Behav. 2009;15(Suppl 1):S1–71.
7. Rodenburg R, Stams GJ, Meijer AM, Aldenkamp AP, Dekovic M. Psychopathology in children with epilepsy: a meta-analysis. J Pediatr Psychol. 2005;30:453–68.
8. Rodenburg R, Meijer AM, Dekovic M, Aldenkamp AP. Family factors and psychopathology in children with epilepsy: a literature review. Epilepsy Behav. 2005;6:488–503.
9. Ramaglia G, Romeo A, Viri M, Lodi M, Sacchi S, Cioffi G. Impact of idiopathic epilepsy on mothers and fathers: strain, burden of care, worries and perception of vulnerability. Epilepsia. 2007;48:1810–3.
10. Valeta T. Psychosocial aspects, parental reactions and needs in idiopathic focal epilepsies. Epileptic Disord. 2016;18:19–22.
11. Valeta T. Impact of epilepsies on women and related psychosocial issues. In: Panayiotopoulos CP, Crawford P, Tomson T, editors. Epilepsies in girls and women, vol. 4. Oxford: Medicinae; 2008. p. 190–7.
12. Manacheril R, Faheem U, Labiner D, Drake K, Chong J. Psychosocial impact of epilepsy in older adults. Healthcare (Basel). 2015;3:1271–83.
13. Cunningham C, Newton R, Appleton R, Hosking G, McKinlay I. Epilepsy—giving the diagnosis. A survey of British paediatric neurologists. Seizure. 2002;11:500–11.
14. World Health Organization. Atlas epilepsy care in the World 2005. Geneva: World Health Organisation; 2005.

# Psychosocial Aspects, Parental Reactions and Needs in Idiopathic (Self-Limited) Focal Epilepsies

24

**Abstract**

This chapter details my research on psychosocial aspects, parental reactions and needs in idiopathic (self-limited) focal epilepsies. This is the first study to provide quantitative and qualitative evidence that idiopathic focal epilepsies have a dramatic impact on parents, with multiple emotional, psychological, social and medical ramifications. The results are based on a questionnaire that I purposely designed and validated and consists of 34 questions, of which 18 are qualitative and 16 quantitative. Unmet negative feelings of panic, fear, and thoughts about death, may affect the parents' reactions and attitude and consequently their parental role, the functioning of their children and the quality of life of the whole family. Practice parameter guidelines for children with idiopathic focal epilepsies that I issued are detailed.

**Keywords**

Questionnaire • Parenting • Attitudes • Fear of death • Guidelines Rolandic epilepsy • Panayiotopoulos syndrome

## What Are the Psychosocial Aspects, Parental Reactions and Needs in Idiopathic Focal Epilepsies?

The psychosocial impact of epilepsy on the affected children and their families has been detailed in Chap. 23. Understandably, attention and research has been primarily focused on severe epilepsies because of profound challenges in

---

Researchers who would like to use Valeta Th. Questionnaire for Parents with Children with Epilepsy© please contact Thalia Valeta at: tvjoyflower@aol.com

© Springer International Publishing AG 2017
T. Valeta, *The Epilepsy Book: A Companion for Patients*,
DOI 10.1007/978-3-319-61679-7_24

dealing with frequent and severe seizures, an endless quest for seizure control and the additional physical, social and psychological problems. The burden placed on the parents of children with idiopathic focal epilepsies (IFE), also known as benign childhood focal epilepsies, has not been emphasized because of the comparatively better prognosis and easier management. Nevertheless, psychological research over the last decade has suggested that in children with IFE parental attitudes and reactions are often severe and contrast with the physician's perception of these epilepsies as uncomplicated and benign conditions [1, 2].

This chapter is to present my recently published research documenting that, despite their excellent prognosis, IFE represent a dramatic experience for the patients and the parents [3]. The parents have significant and unmet needs that may affect the quality of their life, their parental role and therefore the functioning of their children and the quality of life of the whole family.

## What Is the Method That I Used?

My personal interest started in 2000, when talking extensively to parents of children with IFE, I was touched, impressed and inspired by their experiences. I realized that they were concerned for many more issues than the seizures themselves and other than those that they were able to discuss with their physician.

Consequently, I designed a questionnaire in order to (a) identify the parents' reactions and needs, (b) identify the parents feelings during and after the seizure, (c) examine the relationship between the parents and their children after the event, (d) how the event has affected their family, and (e) its impact on the child's health, development and future. The initial questionnaire with the response of 15 parents of children with IFE in St. Thomas' hospital was published in 2005 [1].

Subsequently, in 2008 I initiated a study on parental reactions and needs of children with epilepsy in general. I modified and translated the questionnaire into Greek. The questionnaire, named 'Valeta Thalia Questionnaire for Parents of children with Epilepsy'©, has been validated and consists of 34 questions, of which 18 are qualitative and 16 quantitative. The questionnaire covers the following themes: (a) Parents' and children's demographic and clinical data, (b) Parental attitude, reaction and feelings during and after the seizures, (c) Parental experience to the medical examination, (d) Impact of seizures on parent-child relationship, (e) Impact of seizures on family, (f) Parental reactions and attitude outside the family, (g) Parental reactions and attitude to antiepileptic drugs, and (h) Parental needs other than medical.

Parents were recruited from the clinical practice at the department of Child Neurology Agia Sophia Children's Hospital in Athens. Children with epilepsy were classified according to the ILEA classifications [4]. Out of 100 parents of children with epilepsy who completed the questionnaire, 22 were parents of children with IFE comprising rolandic epilepsy, Panayiotopoulos syndrome and late onset childhood occipital epilepsy of Gastaut.

For analysis of the open ended questions descriptive statistics were used (e.g. means, standard deviation, frequency, % cumulative frequency). Data from the qualitative questions were processed via content analysis methods. The parents' answers (raw data) were summarised in higher order themes in order to provide, in a more parsimonious manner, the participants' behaviour, reaction, and feelings, before, during and after a seizure. Reliability and internal consistency were 0.73 as measured using Cronbach's alpha, with inter-item correlations of 0.379, and corrected item total correlations of 0.355. The participants were given the opportunity to provide more than one answer in order to portray their experiences and express their feelings.

## What Are the Results of My Study?

The responses of the parents of children with IFE to the questionnaire provide interesting material on social and psychological issues. 25% of parents react to the seizures of their children in ways that are not recommended, or are potentially harmful, such as putting a spoon into the child's mouth, give the child a bath, or lifting the child from the floor. Parents had discussed the seizures with their child and the extended family more than with friends or at school to protect their children from bullying at school, or from social stigma. Half of the parents say that their behaviour towards the child has changed. They have become overprotective and less demanding in school performance. Some parent child relationships have become closer and some have not changed.

The following results from 6 representative questions indicate the parental reactions and feelings during and after the seizures, the effect that the seizures have on their everyday life, and finally the parental needs of children with IFE. All the percentages are based on the answers/responses of the parents and not on the number of the parents/participants.

## Feelings of Parents During the Seizure

Negative feelings: Fear, panic, terror 37.5%, Bad 15.6%, Anxiety 9.4%, Insecurity 28.1%, Guilt 3.1%, thoughts about death 6.3%, Calm 3.1%, Denial 3.1%.

For this question, the results are dramatic because the feelings of nearly all the parents during the seizure are negative.

## Feelings of Parents After the Seizure

Negative feelings: Panic, fear, terror 34%, Anxiety 31%, Disappointment 31.8%.
Positive feelings: joy 45%.
Neutral feelings: Secure under the doctor's care, 9.1%.
Denial was expressed by 9.1%.

For this question panic, anxiety, disappointment, dominate. Some, experience joy and relief. The high percentage of joy and relief is because of the attack ending and the child recovering.

During and after the event we notice, parents expressing denial, as an attitude to the problem, which may come from extreme fear.

Figure 24.1 shows the results on the question: Has the event influenced you in the following areas? Figure 24.2 shows the results on the question: How long has this lasted? years, months, weeks? The event has affected parents mostly in that they are scared, their sleep and quality of work was affected (Fig. 24.1) mostly for months, for some years, or weeks (Fig. 24.2).

Figure 24.3 shows the results on the question: Do you need help other than medical?

Figure 24.4 shows the results on the question: Do you need help in any of the following areas?

The parents need help other than medical attention (Fig. 24.3) and specifically education on epilepsies, psychological support for the child, parental support and advocacy groups and psychological support for themselves (Fig. 24.4).

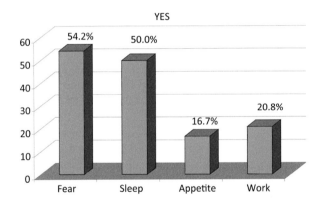

**Fig. 24.1**  Results for the question: "Has the event influenced you in the following areas?"

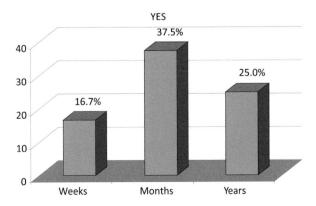

**Fig. 24.2**  Results for the question: "How long has this lasted? years, months, weeks"

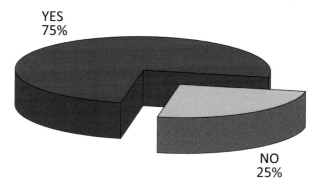

**Fig. 24.3** Results for the question: "Do you need help other than medical?"

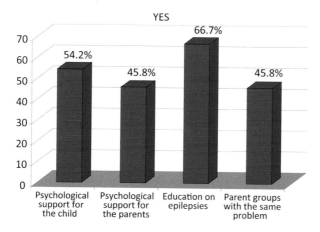

**Fig. 24.4** Results for the question: "Do you need help in any of the following areas?"

## What Is the Significance of This Study?

This is the first study to provide quantitative and qualitative evidence that IFE has a dramatic impact on parents, with multiple emotional, psychological, social and medical ramifications. As the results of this study show, this impact is much more severe than one would expect from a benign and self-limited condition.

Unmet negative feelings of panic, fear, and thoughts about death, as mentioned in the results section, may affect the parents' reactions and attitude and consequently their parental role, the functioning of their children and the quality of life of the whole family. Thus, it is crucial that parents are given sufficient time and opportunity to discuss their concerns with the specialists.

I suggest that practice parameter guidelines for children with IFE and supportive family management and education should be issued:

1. Parents should be given general information about IFE and training to remain calm and confident about their children's condition. Demonstrations of first aid practices for seizures are necessary.
2. Educating parents about epilepsies and different types of seizure will help to alleviate the social stigma surrounding these conditions, which parents often pass on to their children.
3. Parents who have watched their child during a seizure, need specific information and psychological support to overcome anxiety, fear and panic and other negative feelings, as detailed in the results of my study. That should be properly addressed from the time of first diagnosis, in order to improve the quality of life of the child and family.
4. Anxiety and fear may result in overprotection, which interferes with parent – child separation and independence. Psychological support will help parents and patients in coping techniques to manage stress, anger, anxiety or self-esteem. It can moderate parental perceptions of the child's illness and the marital strain related to the child's rearing, thus contribute to effective parenting.

I hope that the results of my study, will assist the patient and parents, inform the physician and, consequently, help to improve the treatment outcome.

## References

1. Valeta T. Parental attitude, reaction and education in benign childhood focal seizures. In: Panayiotopoulos CP, editor. The epilepsies: seizures, syndromes and management. Oxford: Bladon Medical Publishing; 2005. p. 258–61.
2. Valeta T. Parental reactions in benign childhood focal seizures. Epilepsia. 2012;53(Supplem 5):222–3.
3. Valeta T. Psychosocial aspects, parental reactions and needs in idiopathic focal epilepsies. Epileptic Disord. 2016;18:19–22.
4. Berg AT, Berkovic SF, Brodie MJ, Buchhalter J, Cross HJ, Van Emde Boas W, et al. Revised terminology and concepts for organization of seizures and epilepsies: report of the ILAE commission on classification and terminology, 2005-2009. Epilepsia. 2010;51:676–85.

# Stigma in Epilepsy and How to Combat It

**25**

### Abstract

From ancient times, people with epilepsy have been viewed with fear, suspicion, and misunderstanding and were subjected to enormous social stigma including punishments such as outcasts and death. Only in the nineteenth century, the scientific concept of epilepsy as a brain disorder became more widely accepted, especially in Europe and the USA, but again patients with epilepsy continued facing significant discrimination. Widespread ignorance, fear, misunderstanding, and stigma contributed to severe legal and social penalties. Society, prejudice, and people's attitudes can influence the quality of life of people with epilepsy. Increasing knowledge about epilepsy by raising awareness and educating about the disorder is a significant factor toward eradicating epilepsy-related stigma.

### Keywords

Discrimination • Bullying • Enacted stigma • Felt stigma • Concealment • Malleus Maleficarum • Epilepsy care

## What Is Stigma and Its Effect in Discrimination?

Stigma literally means a mark that may be congenital (birth mark), the result of a specific disease, injury, or purposely made either by the individual as means of decoration or others as means of identification.

The actual meaning of stigma in social terms is

- A mark of infamy or disgrace; sign of moral blemish; stain or reproach caused by dishonorable conduct; reproachful characterization (Webster dictionary).
- A distinguishing personal trait that is perceived as or actually is physically, socially, or psychologically disadvantageous (Free Online Medical Dictionary).

The origin of stigma is probably from the Greek word **στίγμα** coming from the Indo-European root **steig** meaning *"to prick" "to stick"* in order to make marks or tattoo somebody for the purpose of identification of usually slaves and prevent their escape. Thus, stigma is a mark separating individuals from one another based on a socially discussed judgment that some persons or groups are tainted and "less than." Stigma often leads to negative beliefs (i.e., stereotypes), the endorsement of those negative stereotypes as real (i.e., prejudice), and a desire to avoid or exclude persons who hold stigmatized statuses (i.e., discrimination). It implies discrimination and prejudice against somebody because of a single or a number of individual features such as illness, health, social status, appearance, age, weight, and education. Of illnesses psychiatric and mental disabilities, epilepsy and AIDS are the most common reasons of stigmatization and discrimination. In order to address the distinctive features of health-related stigma and the social burden of illness, Health-related stigma is defined as a social process or related personal experience characterized by exclusion, rejection, blame, or devaluation that results from experience or reasonable anticipation of an adverse social judgment about a person or group identified with a particular health problem [1].

## Stigma and Discrimination in Epilepsy

*"The history of epilepsy can be summarised as 4000 years of ignorance, superstition, and stigma followed by 100 years of knowledge, superstition, and stigma. Knowing that seizures result from sudden, excessive, abnormal electrical discharges of a set of neurones in the brain, has done little to dispel misunderstanding about epilepsy in most of the world. More than three quarters of sufferers remain untreated, despite the availability in phenobarbitone, of a cheap antiepileptic drug. Epilepsy remains a hidden disease associated with discrimination in the work place, school, and home". (Kale 1997)* [2]

Epilepsy is often surrounded by prejudice and myths. The epilepsy-related stigma has a long ancestry. Some historical outlines may help understand its origins. From the earliest times of civilization, many misconceptions about the condition were conveyed based on the culture of a particular era or in a particular part of the world. People with epilepsy were being looked upon as "being chosen" or as "being possessed" and epilepsy as a "drowning" or "burning" disease depending on the popular belief of that moment or place, with subsequent consequences for treatment and for the attitudes in that society, toward people with epilepsy. In other words people were mystified by epilepsy, and by the seizures which can be sudden or dramatic often with bizarre behavioural and physical symptoms and convulsions.

Unfortunately, for many centuries; people with epilepsy have been viewed with fear, suspicion, and misunderstanding and were subjected to enormous social stigma including punishments such as outcasts and death. For example, epileptic seizures are described as characteristic features to identify witches in *Malleus Maleficarum* (1486), a judicial handbook of witch-hunting written by two Dominican friars under papal authority that lead to persecution, torture, and death of more than 200,000 women in over 300 years.

Only in the nineteenth century, the scientific concept of epilepsy as a brain disorder became more widely accepted, especially in Europe and the USA, but again patients with epilepsy continued facing significant discrimination. Widespread ignorance, fear, misunderstanding, and stigma contributed to severe legal and social penalties.

In Germany, during the Third Reich, a "Law for the Prevention of Offspring with Hereditary Diseases" came into effect in 1934 forcing compulsory sterilization and extermination of people with hereditary disabilities. Epilepsy was included as a "hereditary falling disease."

People with epilepsy were the victims of eugenic sterilization programs in Sweden (1935–1975), many states of the USA (until 1956), and were not allowed to marry (in the UK until 1970).

In many poor-resource countries, around 35 million patients have no access to appropriate treatment either because services are non-existent or because epilepsy is not viewed as a medical problem or a treatable brain disorder but it is still believed that it is related to witchcraft, evil spirits, or sorcery and that the disease is contagious. In some societies the fear of "contamination" by the breath, blood, sperm, and genital secretion of people with epilepsy, and who are not treated, leads to unacceptable responses such as rushing away from a person experiencing a seizure without offering any help. Children with epilepsy, often face discrimination and isolation at school, resulting in low self-esteem and underachievement [3]. Surveys conducted in schools revealed a high rate of social withdrawal among children with epilepsy [4].

The global burden of epilepsy, includes physical hazards resulting from the unpredictability of seizures, social exclusion as a result of negative attitudes of others toward people with epilepsy and the stigma, as children with epilepsy may be banned from school, adults may be barred from marriage, and employment is often denied, even when seizures would not render the work unsuitable or unsafe [5].

The stigmatizing nature of epilepsy and its associated psychopathology in people with epilepsy has been well established. In one recent study of more than 6000 adults from ten European countries, almost half had difficulty accepting their illness, and 17% felt stigmatized by it [6]. Factors predictive of stigma that varied among countries and cultures, included seizure frequency, duration of epilepsy, seizure type, and knowledge of epilepsy. Increasing knowledge about epilepsy by raising awareness and educating about the disorder is a significant factor toward eradicating epilepsy-related stigma.

Society, prejudice, and people's attitudes can influence the quality of life of people with epilepsy.

## Combating Stigma of Epilepsy

To combat stigma and discrimination, it is important to differentiate between enacted and felt stigma.

## What Is Enacted Stigma?

Enacted stigma implies actual episodes of discrimination, both formal and informal, against people with epilepsy solely on the grounds of their having epilepsy [7].

Based on centuries of stigmatization, people with epilepsy experience violations and restrictions of their civil (unequal access to health and life insurance, educational, occupational, and even marital limitations) and human rights (social ostracism) across the world [4]. These violations are more evident in developing countries, but they are also frequently encountered in developed countries with a high profile of civil rights and anti-discrimination laws.

## What Is Felt Stigma and the Consequences of Concealment?

Felt stigma is the personal shame of being epileptic and the fear of encountering enacted stigma [7]. Felt stigma is the main reason that patients with epilepsy often prefer to conceal their condition in order to avoid the consequences of enacted stigma (see Chap. 19 "Metamyth"©/Dramatherapy). This issue of shame and concealment may extend beyond the individual with epilepsy to the entire family and there are many examples where patients with epilepsy are kept at home and their condition kept secret.

Concealment may reduce the likelihood of epilepsy-related discrimination but increases the stress of continuously hiding their condition with the fear that this "secret" may be revealed and adverse treatment, legal and social implications. Thus concealment may impose a far more disruptive effect on their lives than the enacted stigma itself.

Conversely, those resisting to concealment may actually face less stigma, experience less social harm, and be better able to cope with any discrimination while at the same time they avoid the life-long hidden distress and unhappiness experienced by people who conceal.

## Efforts to Combat Stigma

Despite some progress made mainly in developed countries and some positive changes worldwide in public attitudes, stigma remains a main hazard in the lives of people with epilepsy. Fear, misunderstanding, and the resulting social stigma and discrimination surrounding epilepsy often force people with this disorder "into the shadows" [4].

In 1997, the International League Against Epilepsy (ILAE) and the International Bureau for Epilepsy (IBE) joined forces with the World Health Organization to establish "Out of the shadows," a Global Campaign Against Epilepsy to these issues [4].

The aim of the Global Campaign Against Epilepsy is to

- Improve prevention, treatment, care, and services for people with epilepsy.
- Facilitate entry into proper treatment and reduce the financial barriers to treatment.
- Educate people with epilepsy and their families who need support to counter prevailing negative stereotypes and reduce their experience of stigma.
- Increase public awareness of epilepsy as both a medical and social disease, which includes eliminating the myths and misinformation about epilepsy that pose threats to the identity, self-esteem, security, and life opportunities of persons with epilepsy.
- Help and encourage governments to meet their obligations to their citizens with epilepsy by improving health, social, and legislative services.
- Encourage proper anti-stigma campaigns.

Campaigns such as the Global Campaign Against Epilepsy are raising the profile of the disorder with governments and their health-system planners and providers.

Epilepsy associations are moving rapidly from the provision of support and information to an increasingly political role, demanding for better services and less discrimination for their members. A number of strategies have been proposed, including providing education and information, advocacy, and increasing the level of contact between people with epilepsy and people without epilepsy [8, 9].

However, as recently analyzed by Pescosolido et al. [10] for mental disorders, it is important to understand "the complexity and disconfirming evidence of the limits of stigma reduction. While the overriding concern and hope lies in the belief that stigma can be eradicated, research on implicit attitudes as well as more general research on socialization and identity theory suggests there will always be a process of 'us' and 'them' at work in interaction." Only programs, where social network ties are sustained, meaningful, interactive, and positive, are likely to have an influence that is not ephemeral. Attempts and means that are troubling, harmful, or otherwise disturbing, may have a negative impact on stigma reduction. If social systems, from welfare office to treatment clinics to political organizations, encode notions of civility, partnership, citizenship rights, and concern, then it will likely lessen the stigma" [10].

It is hoped that the end result will be a supportive environment in which people with epilepsy can live a good quality of life and retain a good sense of self instead of being wholly defined by one's illness. The success of a number of cases and initiatives suggests that this is possible.

While you can't stop all teasing, no child should be afraid to go to school or face humiliation or cruelty. Unfortunately, children with disabilities are more likely to face bullying. It is important to be aware of it, encourage your child to talk about it, and work with teachers to prevent it. Bullying can lead to depression, physical problems such as headaches and poor appetite, absences from school and even suicidal thoughts. The U.S. Department of Health and Human Services' Stop!' campaign has information on what kids and adults can do.

## Recommended Readings

- Atlas: epilepsy care in the World 2005. World Health Organisation, Geneva. In http://www.who.int/mental_health/neurology/Epilepsy_atlas_r1.pdf
- Epilepsy: Stigma and Management in http://scialert.net/fulltext/?doi=crn.2011.1.14&org=10
- Confronting the stigma of epilepsy in https://www.ncbi.nlm.nih.gov/pmc/articles/PMC3200035/
- Epilepsy and bullying in: http://www.youngepilepsy.org.uk/about-epilepsy/living-with-epilepsy/epilepsy-and-its-impact-on-children/epilepsy-and-bullying.html
- Stop Bulling now in: http://stopbullyingnow.com/.
- Malleus Maleficarum in: http://www.malleusmaleficarum.org/downloads/MalleusAcrobat.pdf

## References

1. Weiss MG, Ramakrishna J. Stigma interventions and research for international health. Lancet. 2006;367:536–8.
2. Kale R. Bringing epilepsy out of the shadows. BMJ. 1997;315:2–3.
3. Valeta T. Impact of newly identified epileptic seizures in patients and family. In: Panayiotopoulos CP, editor. Newly identified epileptic seizures: diagnosis, procedures and management, vol. 3. Oxford: Medicinae; 2007. p. 138–44.
4. World Health Organization. Atlas epilepsy care in the world 2005. Geneva: World Health Organisation; 2005.
5. de Boer HM. Epilepsy stigma: moving from a global problem to global solutions. Seizure. 2010;19:630–6.
6. Baker GA. People with epilepsy: what do they know and understand, and how does this contribute to their perceived level of stigma? Epilepsy Behav. 2002;3:26–32.
7. Scambler G. Health-related stigma. Sociol Health Illn. 2009;31:441–55.
8. Valeta T, de Boer HM. Stigma and discrimination in epilepsy. In: Panayiotopoulos CP, editor. Atlas of epilepsies. London: Springer; 2010. p. 1363–6.
9. de Boer HM, Mula M, Sander JW. The global burden and stigma of epilepsy. Epilepsy Behav. 2008;12:540–6.
10. Pescosolido BA, Martin JK, Lang A, Olafsdottir S. Rethinking theoretical approaches to stigma: a framework integrating normative influences on stigma (FINIS). Soc Sci Med. 2008;67:431–40.

# Websites and Other Resources for People with Epilepsy

**Abstract**

One of the most important recommendations made in this book, is that patients and parents should learn as much as possible about their specific type of epilepsy, appropriate management, safety and quality of life. This is even more important today in a patient-physician shared-decision making environment. Recently, there has been an explosive growth of the Internet and Web as tools for seeking and communicating health and medical information about epilepsy. This chapter provides information about the best websites and other resources for people with epilepsy.

**Keywords**

Epilepsy guidelines • Epilepsy practice parameters • International League against epilepsy • Epilepsy Bureau for epilepsy • PubMed Bookshelf • Epilepsy society • Epilepsy action • American epilepsy society • American epilepsy foundation • Epilepsy e-communities • Epilepsy organizations

## Recommendations

My recommendations for people with epilepsy and their families is to get the maximal information possible for their problem

- Is it an epileptic seizure or something else?
- Is the diagnosis of epileptic seizures firmly established?
- What type of epilepsy is this?
- What are the needed safety measures and means of preventing seizures?

- What are the social, educational, employment and other implications?
- What is the best AED and at what dose if this is needed?
- What are the side effects of drugs?
- What other non-epileptic symptoms or diseases can happen, how to prevent or treat them

Get involved in epilepsy communities and shared your experience with other patients who have the same epilepsy type as you.

## The Web Provides Significant Information and Allows Important Communication Amongst People with Epilepsy

There has been an explosive growth of the Internet and Web as tools for seeking and communicating health and medical information. An increasing number of physicians and patients use Web search engines to seek very detailed advice and solicit or share specific medical and health information. More specialized medical or health websites are now available.

There is a rapid growth in the literature addressing the role of the Internet in medicine and in particular patient education, patient support networks, education and communication among health providers, and communication between providers and patients.

In this shared-decision-making medical environment, immediate access to such information has been of great benefit to health-care professionals and patients. However, there is growing concern that a substantial proportion of clinical information on the Web might be inaccurate, erroneous, misleading, or fraudulent, and thereby pose a threat to public health. Medical website quality is being tested through many sources and guidelines for quality criteria are being developed. With e-mail use patients also have easy, direct and fast access to experts around the world. Parents and patients often use the wide information provided on the Internet for formulating their own opinion regarding diagnosis and management. They are entitled to do so and this is often useful.

## Important Epilepsy Books with Free of Access

The following books on epilepsy are available charge free to professionals and public. They are written mainly for health care professionals but they are also a useful and reliable reading for patients and their relatives. They are particularly important in regard to the diagnosis of specific types of epilepsy such as epileptic syndromes as well as for the various treatments.

**The PubMed Bookshelf of the National Center for Biotechnology Information** (**NCBI**) enables users to easily browse, retrieve, and read content, and spurs discovery of related information for epilepsy. http://www.ncbi.nlm.nih.gov/books?term=epilepsy

The Epilepsies: Seizures, Syndromes and Management.
Panayiotopoulos CP.
Oxfordshire (UK): Bladon Medical Publishing; 2005.
Imitators of Epilepsy. 2nd edition.
Kaplan PW, Fisher RS, editors.
New York: Demos Medical Publishing; 2005.
An Introduction to Epilepsy [Internet].
Bromfield EB, Cavazos JE, Sirven JI, editors.
West Hartford (CT): American Epilepsy Society; 2006.
Effectiveness and Safety of Antiepileptic Medications in Patients With Epilepsy [Internet].
Talati R, Scholle JM, Phung OJ, et al.
Rockville (MD): Agency for Healthcare Research and Quality (US); 2011 Dec. (Comparative Effectiveness Reviews, No. 40.)
Transient Loss of Consciousness ('Blackouts') Management in Adults and Young People [Internet].
National Clinical Guideline Centre for Acute and Chronic Conditions (UK).
London: Royal College of Physicians (UK); 2010 Aug. (NICE Clinical Guidelines, No. 109.)
Jasper's Basic Mechanisms of the Epilepsies [Internet]. 4th edition.
Noebels JL, Avoli M, Rogawski MA, et al., editors.
Bethesda (MD): National Center for Biotechnology Information (US); 2012.
GeneReviews™ [Internet].
Pagon RA, Bird TD, Dolan CR, et al., editors.
Seattle (WA): University of Washington, Seattle; 1993.

**From channels to commissioning—a practical guide to epilepsy** is the 15th edition of the lecture notes of the material used in the biannual epilepsy teaching weekend organized under the auspices of the UK Chapter of the International League against Epilepsy. It can be found in the website of the Epilepsy Society UK.

https://www.epilepsysociety.org.uk/lecture-notes-0#.WIfGMfmLTIU

There are 59 chapters (which can be downloaded in pdf) including topics such as

- Genetics of the epilepsies
- Psychiatric disorders in epilepsy
- Epilepsy and sleep
- Neuropsychology—testing the brain
- Non-pharmacological treatments for epilepsy: the case for and against complementary and alternative medicines
- Psychosocial outcome
- Epilepsy and learning disability
- Employment
- Driving
- Epilepsy and the law
- Medico-legal aspects of epilepsy

- Provision of clinical services for people with epilepsy
- The role of the voluntary organizations in epilepsy
- Social work support in the community

**"Epilepsy diagnosis" manual** is an excellent source for information about seizures and syndromes from the ILAE Commission on Classification and Terminology of the International League against Epilepsy. The goal of epilepsydiagnosis.org is to make available, in an easy to understand form, latest concepts relating to seizures and the epilepsies. The principle goal is to assist clinicians who look after people with epilepsy anywhere in the world to diagnose seizure type(s), diagnose epilepsy syndromes and define the aetiology of the epilepsy. https://www.epilepsydiagnosis.org/.

## Guidelines and Practice Parameters

The following are guidelines and practice parameters for epilepsy. These are mainly for health care professionals but they are also extremely helpful for patients who may wish an in-depth study of their health.

## ILAE Guidelines

http://www.ilae.org/Visitors/Centre/Guidelines.cfm

- Management
- Pediatric/Obstetric
- AEDs
- Treatment other than AEDs
- Diagnosis
- Other Guidelines & Reports
- Creating Guidelines
- Archive
- The current state of epilepsy guidelines (December 2015)

## American Epilepsy Society

http://www.aesnet.org/go/practice/guidelines

These practice parameters and guidelines related to the care and treatment of epilepsy are developed collaboratively between the American Epilepsy Society and the American Academy of Neurology.

All guideline files are in pdf format.

- Evidence-Based Guideline: Treatment of Convulsive Status Epilepticus in Children and Adults: Report of the Guideline Committee of the American Epilepsy Society
- New Guideline for Treatment of Prolonged Seizures in Children and Adults
- A treatment algorithm that comprises three phases of treatment
- Evidence-based Guideline: Management of First Unprovoked Seizure in Adults
  Evidence-based Guideline: Vagus nerve stimulation for the treatment of epilepsy

## Practice Parameters

- Practice Parameter update: Management issues for women with epilepsy—Focus on pregnancy: Obstetrical complications and change in seizure frequency
- Practice Parameter update: Management issues for women with epilepsy—Focus on pregnancy: Vitamin K, folic acid, blood levels, and breastfeeding
- Practice Parameter update: Management issues for women with epilepsy—Focus on pregnancy: Teratogenesis and perinatal outcomes
- Practice Parameter: Treatment of the child with a first unprovoked seizure
- Practice Parameter: Diagnostic assessment of the child with status epilepticus
- Practice Parameter: Evaluating an apparent unprovoked first seizure in adults
- Practice Parameter: Temporal lobe and localized neocortical resections for epilepsy

## Additional Papers

- Antiepileptic Drug Selection for People with HIV/AIDS
- Treatment of New Onset Epilepsy
- Treatment of Refractory Epilepsy
- Use of serum prolactin in diagnosing epileptic seizures
- Other AAN Epilepsy Guidelines and Practice Parameters

## NICE (National Institute of Clinical Excellence) U.K.

In the UK, the NICE (National Institute of Clinical Excellence) has recently updated the relevant guidelines and recommendations for children and adults with epilepsy.

The epilepsies: the diagnosis and management of the epilepsies in adults and children in primary and secondary care in http://www.nice.org.uk/nicemedia/live/13635/57779/57779.pdf

The diagnosis and management of epilepsy in children, young people and adults (booklet for patients and carers) http://guidance.nice.org.uk/CG137/PublicInfo/doc/English

## Epilepsy: Clinical Case Scenarios

Clinical case scenarios are an educational and learning resource designed to improve and assess users' knowledge of the epilepsies and its application in primary and secondary care. The resource is available in a PDF document for individual learning or as a power point presentation to help facilitate group learning.

The clinical case scenarios illustrate how the recommendations from the epilepsies can be applied to the care of patients presenting to primary and secondary care
    http://guidance.nice.org.uk/CG137/ClinicalScenarios

- CG137 Epilepsy: clinical case scenarios—adults: PDF
- CG137 Epilepsy: clinical case scenarios—adults: Powerpoint
- CG137 Epilepsy: clinical case scenarios—children and young people: PDF
- CG137 Epilepsy: clinical case scenarios—children and young people: Powerpoint

## Scottish Intercollegiate Guidelines Network (SIGN)

The Scottish Intercollegiate Guidelines Network (SIGN) provides significant information and guidelines for adults and children with epilepsy.

### SIGN Guideline 143: Diagnosis and Management of Epilepsy in Adults

www.sign.ac.uk/guidelines/fulltext/143/index.html

## Significant Epilepsy Organizations

### International League Against Epilepsy (ILAE)

http://www.ilae.org/
    The International League Against Epilepsy (ILAE) is the official organization of epilepsy health care professional. The goals of the ILAE are:

- To advance and disseminate knowledge about epilepsy
- To promote research, education and training
- To improve services and care for patients, especially by prevention, diagnosis and treatment

**Important Sections to Look at Are: Guidelines & Resource Center**
http://www.ilae.org/Visitors/Centre/Index.cfm
The International League Against Epilepsy's Resource Center is the gateway for comprehensive information about the condition of epilepsy.

- **Guidelines & Reports**—Current practice guidelines, reports, and position papers
- **Books on Epilepsy**—listing of books published that are relevant to epilepsy
- **Links to Epilepsy Organizations**—Links to related professional organizations, International Bureau and national chapters, epilepsy foundations and other National Government Organizations, governmental health related departments and organizations, and other sites of potential interest
- **EEG Machines**—Bulletin board showing hospitals in need of equipment and those who are upgrading who could donate or sell used equipment.
- **Epilepsy Bibliography—Books and Monographs (EBBM)**—A searchable reference list of epilepsy-related books and monographs published in the world since 1945.
- **Worldwide Epilepsy Resource Directory**—A comprehensive database of epilepsy-related resources from around the world

## Education

http://www.ilae.org/Visitors/Centre/EDUIndex.cfm
The International League Against Epilepsy's mission is to ensure that health professionals, patients and their care providers, governments, and the public worldwide have the educational and research resources that are essential in understanding, diagnosing and treating persons with epilepsy. Education is a focal point of ILAE activities, including ILAE Congresses worldwide and distance education.

Diagnostic Manual, VIREPA, Regional Educational Activities, Non-ILAE Educational Resources, Videos

## Epilepsy Care

The ILAE provides some resources that can be useful to medical personnel caring for persons with epilepsy.

- Worldwide AED Database– This database lists the various formulations and preparations of drugs available to treat epilepsy by country, brand and generic name.

- ILAE Classification and Terminology Report – View reports, translations, and other tools, as well as other information about the Classification & Terminology Commission
- Diagnostic Methods Commission
- Genetics Commission
- Pediatrics Commission
- Therapeutics Commission

The ILAE organisation consists of 114 national chapters. To find information for individual ILAE Chapters around the world (address, contact numbers, persons involved, activities) go to http://www.ilae.org/Visitors/Chapters/chapter-select.cfm and select the country that you are interested for.

## The International Bureau for Epilepsy (IBE)

http://www.ibe-epilepsy.org/

The International Bureau for Epilepsy (IBE) is an organisation of laypersons and professionals interested in the medical and non-medical aspects of epilepsy. The IBE addresses such social problems as education, employment, insurance, driving licence restrictions and public awareness.

The International Bureau for Epilepsy provides assistance by offering international support, by creating means for worldwide exchange of information and, where possible, by setting standards which provide an international policy focus and identity for all persons with epilepsy. Much of this work is accomplished through the IBE working commissions, composed of volunteers who are experts in their subjects.

To improve international understanding of epilepsy, IBE publishes a quarterly magazine, the International Epilepsy News, which keeps readers informed on international developments. In addition, IBE publishes a comprehensive range of reports and information booklets covering a wide range of subjects, including education, employment, insurance, driving regulations and self-help groups. For further information please go to the Publications section on http://www.ibe-epilepsy.org/publications. Many of these publications in various languages (English, French, Portuguese, Spanish, Mandarin and Cantonese Chinese, Italian, German, Dutch, Turkish, Greek, Russian) are available for automatic download.

- Traveller's Handbook for People with Epilepsy
- Employing People with Epilepsy—Principles for Good Practice
- Live Beyond Epilepsy—Be Inspired
- Future in Mind Report
- Annual Reports
- Epilepsy and Employment: a guide for workers and employers
- IBE History: 50 years—Focused on Epilepsy—August 1, 2011
- Epilepsy in the WHO—Fostering Epilepsy Care in Europe
- Epilepsy in the WHO South East Asian Region—Bridging the gap

- Epilepsy in the Western Pacific Region: Call to Action
- African Region: Bridging the gap
- Epilepsy in the Eastern Mediterranean Region—Bridging the gap
- Informe sobre la Epilepsia en Latinoamérica
- Epilepsy in North America
- PAHO Strategic Plan for Epilepsy

## World Health Organisation

http://www.who.int/topics/epilepsy/en/
See also: Global Campaign against Epilepsy: Out of the Shadows http://www.who.int/mental_health/management/globalepilepsycampaign/en/index.html and obtain free of charge the pdf of "Atlas: Epilepsy care in the world 2005" http://www.who.int/mental_health/neurology/Epilepsy_atlas_r1.pdf
The CREST Study
Collaborative Research on Epilepsy Stigma Project
Developing Approaches to Reducing Stigma of Epilepsy

## Epilepsy Websites in UK, USA, Canada and Australia

### United Kingdom

### Epilepsy Society
http://www.epilepsysociety.org.uk/
Provides up to date information on all aspects of living with epilepsy, from driving, employment and pregnancy to leisure, travel and medication.
Helplines usually offers callers:

- up-to-date information
- an opportunity to speak to trained and experienced staff
- informal counselling
- emotional support
- written resources as available and appropriate
- referrals to other agencies/bodies
- a caller-led service
- respectful listening
- a call-back service to anybody who has financial difficulties and who cannot afford the call.

Information includes:

- Healthcare professionals involved in my care
- Seizures—why they happen

- Triggers for seizures
- Treatment options for seizures
- Managing my epilepsy
- Day to day needs for people with epilepsy
- Driving regulations
- Work and epilepsy
- Safety and epilepsy
- Alcohol, drugs and epilepsy
- Risks with epilepsy
- What women need to know
- What next?
- Long term conditions
- Sex, relationships and education
- Connecting with others
- Your feelings about epilepsy
- Coming to terms with epilepsy

### Epilepsy Action

http://www.epilepsy.org.uk/

Epilepsy Action is the largest member-led epilepsy organization in Britain. As well as campaigning to improve epilepsy services and raise awareness of the condition, they offer assistance to people in a number of ways including a national network of branches, accredited volunteers, regular regional conferences and freephone and email helplines.

Epilepsy Action Head Office:

New Anstey House, Gate Way Drive, Yeadon, LEEDS, LS19 7XY, United Kingdom

Phone: 0113 210 8800 Fax: 0113 391 0300 Email: epilepsy@epilepsy.org.uk

Freephone Helpline: 0808 800 5050 International Callers: +44 113 210 8850 Email Helpline: helpline@epilepsy.org.uk Text Helpline: 0753 741 0044

Epilepsy action supports people with epilepsy through

- freephone telephone helpline,
- email helpline,
- text message helpline
- Twitter helpline
- local branches throughout the UK,
- online community,
- conferences for people with epilepsy and their families,
- accredited volunteers,
- Sapphire epilepsy specialist nurse scheme

Publications and video information to anyone interested in epilepsy, in the form of

- leaflets,
- factsheets,
- booklets,
- videos,
- CD and audiobooks,
- ID cards and seizure diaries.

Their website provides information for

- young people,
- children,
- parents,
- older people, and
- the media;
- general information like first aid for seizures; and
- facts, figures and terminology.

They campaign to raise standards of care through contact with doctors, nurses, social workers, government and other organizations,

- improve the support for children and young people with epilepsy in education
- give people with epilepsy a fair chance of finding and keeping a job,
- raise awareness of epilepsy and first aid for seizures

Leaflets that can be loaded as PDF files include:

- The basics
  Introduction to epilepsy, seizures, first aid
- Treatment
  Epilepsy medicines, treatments, healthcare
- Help and support
  Helpline services, benefits, travel to work
- People with epilepsy
  Particular groups of people
- The law
  Driving, Equality Act
- Diagnosis
  How it happens
- Living with epilepsy
  Safety, sports, caring for children, travel
- Health matters
  Memory, stress, bone health
- Education and work
  Education, exams, epilepsy at work

- Epilepsy syndromes
  Some specific childhood epilepsies

## Epilepsy Research UK
http://www.epilepsyresearch.org.uk/
  Epilepsy Research UK provides a. research grants specifically for all aspects of epilepsy and b. significant information about this condition that can be downloaded as pdf files

- About epilepsy
- Causes of epilepsy
- Diagnosis of epilepsy
- Treatments for epilepsy
- Epilepsy & Family Planning
- Childhood epilepsy syndromes
- Sudden unexpected death in epilepsy
- Videos about epilepsy research
- Other sources of information
- Information Leaflets

  Information leaflets include:

What is epilepsy
Epilepsy checklist
Epilepsy and photosensitivity
What to do when someone has a seizure
Recording seizures
Diagnosing Epilepsy

  Risk and safety

Epilepsy and driving
Epilepsy and safety in leisure activities
Epilepsy and safety in sport
Epilepsy and safety at work
Epilepsy and safety in school, college and university
Epilepsy and safety in the home

  Treatments for epilepsy
  Epilepsy and anti-malarial medication
  FAQs on anti-epileptic drugs
  Anti-epileptic drugs
  Treatments for epilepsy

## Support Groups for Parents of Children with Some Types of Syndrome in the UK

In the UK there are support groups for parents of children with some types of syndrome. Details of the support groups can be obtained from the following:

**Contact A Family**
209-211 City Road
London EC1V 1JN
Telephone: +44 (0)20 7608 8714
Freephone helpline: +44 (0)808 808 3555
Email: info@cafamily.org.uk, https://www.cafamily.org.uk/

## Young Epilepsy

http://www.youngepilepsy.org.uk/
Epilepsy Helpline: 01342 831342
Residential care

## Epilepsy Scotland

http://www.epilepsyscotland.org.uk/
Epilepsy Scotland Helpline: 0808 800 2200
Helpline email: helpline@epilepsyscotland.org.uk
Helpline text: 0808 800 2200

All guides are excellent and can be downloaded free of charge as pdf files and these include:

Epilepsy explained
Guide to Epilepsy and Occupational Health
(Epilepsy and Occupational Health, aimed at employers)
A Women's Guide to Epilepsy
(For every woman affected by epilepsy)
An Employers Guide to Epilepsy
(What would you do if one of your employees told you they had epilepsy?)
Brian learns about Epilepsy
(For pre-school children whose parent has epilepsy)
Diagnosing Epilepsy
(Step by step explanation of an epilepsy diagnosis)
Emotional Wellbeing Guide
(This guide will help you understand how your epilepsy may effect your emotional wellbeing)
Epilepsy and Driving
(Important information on driving regulations for anyone with epilepsy)
Epilepsy and Employment
(Find out your rights and responsibilities at work)
Epilepsy and Later Life
(Information for anyone affected by epilepsy in later life)

Epilepsy and Leisure
(Keeping leisure and sports activities safe)
Teenage Guide
(An Epilepsy guide to getting on with your life, suitable for 13–19 year olds)
Epilepsy and Memory
(Explaining why people with epilepsy often experience memory problems and why can be done to help)
(A summary of all treatments currently available for people with epilepsy)
Farah and Ted visit the hospital
(For pre-school/early primary school children going through diagnosis)
First Aid for Seizures
(Useful step by step first aid to hand to friends, family and colleagues)
Epilepsy—a Guide for Teachers
(Everything a teacher needs to know about epilepsy)
Seizures Explained
(An overview of different types of seizures)
Staying Safe with Epilepsy
(Essential guide for keeping safe, often used by occupational therapy/social work for assessments)
Living with epilepsy
(Inspiring personal stories from people affected by epilepsy)
Factsheets
(Helpful factsheets about epilepsy)
Get answers: A to Z Glossary
(Learn more about terms associated with epilepsy)
There are also Podcasts/DVD's from team members

## SUDEP Action

http://www.patient.co.uk/support/Epilepsy-Bereaved.htm
Tel: 01235 772 850 Bereavement Contact Line: 01235 772 852
SUDEP Action is dedicated to raising awareness of epilepsy risks and tackling epilepsy deaths including Sudden Unexpected Death in Epilepsy. It is the only UK charity specialised in supporting and involving people bereaved by epilepsy.
Their services include bereavement support, counselling, help with understanding the inquest process and in collaboration with UK research teams, the involvement of bereaved families and professionals in research through the Epilepsy Deaths Register.
They offer:

- Someone to listen
- A confidential service
- Opportunities to speak with someone who has personal experience of an epilepsy death
- Information about epilepsy deaths and SUDEP
- Meetings with other families bereaved through epilepsy
- A regular magazine

If you have lost a loved one to epilepsy, please contact their bereavement support line. The team offer support and information which could help.

## United States of America

### Epilepsy Foundation
http://www.epilepsyfoundation.org/index.cfm
   **Mailing Address:**
   Epilepsy Foundation, 8301 Professional Place East, Suite 200, Landover, MD 20785-7223
   **Telephone:** 1-800-332-1000
   Spanish Language Service (Spanish Speakers Only): 1-866-748-8008
   The Epilepsy Foundation of America® is the national voluntary agency dedicated solely to the welfare of the people with epilepsy in the U.S. and their families. The organization works to ensure that people with seizures are able to participate in all life experiences; to improve how people with epilepsy are perceived, accepted and valued in society; and to promote research for a cure. In addition to programs conducted at the national level, epilepsy clients throughout the United States are served by 48 Epilepsy Foundation affiliates around the country.
   Typical of the Foundation's national programs are its Jeanne A. Carpenter Epilepsy Legal Defense Fund, the H.O.P.E. (Helping Other People with Epilepsy) Mentoring Program, a Public Policy Institute, Seniors' and Women's Health Initiatives, the Kids Speak Up! advocacy program, a school personnel training program, outreach to youth and to the Hispanic community, employment programs and a research grants program. Services commonly provided in local communities are

- information and referral,
- counseling,
- patient and family advocacy,
- school and community education,
- support groups and
- camps for children.

Its website, www.epilepsyfoundation.org, offers a comprehensive, medically approved consumer information about epilepsy and seizures on the Internet for people who seek information about epilepsy.
   The following are examples of the information provided at the Website:

**Start Here!**
- About Epilepsy
- Diagnosis
- Treatment
- Find a Doctor
- Living With Epilepsy
- Local Affiliate

**For…**
- Parents & Caregivers
- Youth & Young Adults
- Seniors
- Women
- Educators
- Advocates

**Resources**
- Epilepsy Resource Center
- First Aid
- Medications
- eNewsletter
- eCommunity
- Driving Laws
- Local Affiliates
- Epilepsy USA Magazine
- Epilepsy In The News
- Newsroom
- Driving and Travel
- Safety
- Epilepsy Legal Defense Fund
- Financial Planning
- Employment Topics
- Veterans
- eNewsletter
- Books, Catalog, etc.
- Healthcare Professionals
- Training

Other Important Resources:

Epilepsy and Seizure Videos, the best and most comprehensive epilepsy content available on the web (video library)

Epileptic Seizures First Aid instructions, a few things you can do to help someone who is having a seizure of any kind

Epilepsy Clinical Trials 101, who is it for, where can I find a clinical trial?

Epilepsy Therapy Pipeline, the pipeline of epilepsy therapies in various stages of development. See what is available and what is coming up.

# Canada

## The Canadian Epilepsy Alliance
The Canadian Epilepsy Alliance is a Canada wide network of grassroots organizations dedicated to the promotion of independence and quality of life for people with

epilepsy and their families, through support services, information, advocacy, and public awareness.

The Canadian Epilepsy Alliance includes rural, urban, local, and provincial incorporated Epilepsy Associations from coast to coast in Canada. An exciting array of epilepsy services is provided by members of the Canadian Epilepsy Alliance from coast to coast, ranging from counseling, education, advocacy and public awareness, to employment help, children's programs, support groups, lending libraries, conferences and special events.

http://www.epilepsymatters.com/english/index.html

http://www.epilepsymatters.com/french/index.html

Detailed Information in English and French is provided in topics such as:

- Explaining Epilepsy
- Diagnosing Epilepsy
- Types of Seizures
- Epilepsy Syndromes
- Photosensitive Epilepsy
- SUDEP
- Psychological and Social Issues
- Behavioural and Emotional Changes in Persons with Epilepsy
- Learning and Behaviour in Children with Epilepsy
- The Impact of Childhood Epilepsy on the Family
- Sex and Epilepsy
- Alcohol and Epilepsy
- Nutrition and Epilepsy
- Driving
- Employment
- Life Insurance
- Safety
- Depression
- Memory Problems
- First Aid For Convulsive Seizures—eg. Tonic Clonic, Grand Mal, Febrile
- First Aid for Non-Convulsive seizures—eg. Absence, Complex Partial
- Treatments for Epilepsy
- Alternative and Complementary Therapies
- Epilepsy Surgery
- Vagus Nerve Stimulation
- Ketogenic Diet

## Australia

### Epilepsy Australia

http://www.epilepsyaustralia.net/

Epilepsy Australia is the national coalition of Australian Epilepsy Associations raising their voices as one to advance the cause of all Australians living with epilepsy.

Actively delivering counseling, support and information to all who access our services, Epilepsy Australia is committed to raising awareness and understanding of the very real issues faced by those living with epilepsy.

The unpredictable nature of seizures can force people to stay at home, fearful of a seizure occurring in public. Would you know what to do if you saw someone having a seizure?

A goal of Epilepsy Australia is for every household in Australia to be seizure aware. Epilepsy Australia member associations provide many services including:

- current information about epilepsy, its treatment and management
- counseling & personal support
- client focused workshops & seminars
- support groups
- recreational programs & weekend retreats
- advocacy & referral services
- community & workplace education
- accredited epilepsy training
- membership benefits

For more information about the services offered by your state or territory association, call the **Epilepsy Australia National Helpline 1300 852 853**

## Epilepsy Australia Affiliates
- Epilepsy ACT
- Epilepsy Association of South Australia & Northern Territory Inc
- Epilepsy Association of Tasmania
- Epilepsy Foundation of Victoria
- Epilepsy Queensland Inc
- Epilepsy Association of Western Australia

**Epilepsy Australia** publishes information of the highest standard on epilepsy and related issues for all members of the community who seek to gain a better understanding of the impact of living with epilepsy.

- Epilepsy Resources
- The Epilepsy Report
- Epifile: an epilepsy management manual
- Epilepsy Information for Indigenous Communities
- Sudden Unexpected Death in Epilepsy
- Collection of Epilepsy Articles
- Epilepsy explained
- Treatment options
- Epilepsy and Risk
- Epilepsy and Lifestyle

Seizure First Aid

- First Aid for seizures occurring in water
- Wheelchair First Aid
- Downloadable First Aid guide

Advocacy
Epilepsy Australia's mission is to actively advocate for people with epilepsy and other seizure disorders where a national outcome is sought.

- Employment
    Epilepsy and the Workplace
- Position Statements
    Epilepsy & Driving

## e-Communities

e-Communities provide the opportunity of people facing issues and concerns about living and dealing with epilepsy to meet and exchange ideas, support and experience. Listed below are websites that offer discussion forums, chat rooms, and other opportunities to allow you to share your experiences and thoughts about epilepsy.
https://www.epilepsyfoundation.org/e-Communities
The e-Communities offer the unique opportunity to interact with individuals affected by epilepsy from around the world through discussion forums and real-time chats. Some specific forums include Parents Helping Parents, Women and Epilepsy, Epilepsy at Work, and Poetry and Prose.
my.epilepsy.com
An online resource to connect with others affected by epilepsy. Read or post your experiences in one of the message boards or participate in a live chat. This site also offers you the opportunity to develop your own blog.
For Teens
www.goeyc.org
This forum offers straight talk for teens about living with epilepsy. It's interactive and inclusive, with links to e-communities and social networking websites. It also offers opportunities to submit personal stories and questions to medical experts.
For Kids
www.abilityonline.org
This is a Canadian-based internet community where kids with disabilities or illness can meet others like them, make friends from all over the world, share their hopes and fears, find role-models and mentors, and feel like they belong.

## Useful Links for Patients

The links below are to non-profit organizations that may be useful for people with epilepsy:

A pediatric healthcare site with information on epilepsy: AboutKidsHealth.ca

The Anita Kaufmann Foundation—www.AKFUS.org

American Association for Intellectual and Developmental Disabilities—www.aaidd.org

Canine Epilepsy Network: http://www.canine-epilepsy.net/

Canine Epilepsy Resources: http://www.canine-epilepsy.com/Resources.html

Center for Disease Control and Prevention—Epilepsy Resources: http://www.cdc.gov/epilepsy/resources.htm

Citizens United for Research in Epilepsy (CURE)—www.CUREepilepsy.orgl.

Danny Did Foundation: http://www.dannydid.org/

Dravet Foundation—www.dravetfoundation.org

Epilepsy Advocate: http://www.epilepsyadvocate.com/resources/epilepsy-programs.aspx

Epilepsy Foundation (EF) and local EF affiliates—www.efa.org

Epilepsy Life Links—www.epilepsylifelinks.com

EpilepsyResource.net:  http://www.epilepsyresource.net/Epilepsy_Information.html

FACES—http://faces.med.nyu.edu/

Hope for Hypothalamic Hamartomas http://hopeforhh.org/

International Dravet Epilepsy Action League http://www.dravet.org or patient-info@dravet.org

Intractable Childhood Epilepsy Alliance http://www.ice-epilepsy.org/

Lennox-Gastaut Syndrome Foundation: www.lgsfoundation.org or info@lgs-foundation.org

Live Beyond Epilepsy: http://www.livebeyondepilepsy.com/resources

My Epilepsy Diary—http://www.epilepsy.com/seizurediary

National Association of Epilepsy Centers: http://www.naec-epilepsy.org/default.htm

Seizure Tracker—www.seizuretracker.com

SEN Teacher Resources: http://www.senteacher.org/Condition/7/Epilepsy.xhtml

US Veterans Affairs: http://www.epilepsy.va.gov/

## Epilepsy Advocate

http://www.epilepsyadvocate.com/

Epilepsy Advocates are people living with epilepsy and caregivers who share their personal success stories online and within local communities. Their purpose is to inspire people to interact with other people with epilepsy, learn from one another, and make positive changes in each other's lives.

Any patient can get involved by joining the community or by signing up to attend an upcoming Epilepsy Advocate community event.

## WebEase

https://www.webease.org/

WebEase stands for **Epilepsy, Awareness, Support, and Education**. It is a free, web-based self-management program for adults with epilepsy.

WebEase encourages you to make decisions that are consistent with your own goals. WebEase doesn't replace instructions from your doctor, but helps you better follow those instructions and gain better control over managing your epilepsy.

With WebEase, adults with epilepsy set goals and create a personal plan to improve or maintain skills, including:

Taking medications as prescribed.

Managing stress.

Getting a good night's sleep.

People can use WebEase to watch videos of others who have dealt with similar issues or read from trusted on-line sources. WebEase also includes MyLog, an online health diary that gives feedback about how their medication schedule, stress, and sleep may be related to their seizures.

Because WebEase adapts to your needs, you only work on the parts that matter to you.

WebEase is for adults with epilepsy who are interested in improving the way they manage their epilepsy. You can use WebEase regardless of where you are in life, or how long you have lived with epilepsy.

## Epilepsy Scholarships

http://www.collegescholarships.org/health/epileptic-students.htm

http://www.excite.com/education/financial-aid/epilepsy-scholarships

Pursuing higher education may be challenging for patients with epilepsy that may also have financial difficulties. To assist students with epilepsy, there are some epilepsy scholarships of which the most popular in USA are:

- Pfizer Epilepsy Scholarship
- Epilepsy Foundation Scholarship Fund
- Elam Baer and Janis Clay Educational Scholarship
- Epilepsy Foundation of Western/Central Pennsylvania
- Epilepsy Foundation of Idaho

# Index

© Springer International Publishing AG 2017
T. Valeta, *The Epilepsy Book: A Companion for Patients*,
DOI 10.1007/978-3-319-61679-7

Printed in the United States
By Bookmasters